Pharmacology of Essential Medicines

AF825604

K. Mukhopadhyay
Prof. and H.O.D.
Department of Pharmacology
College of Medicine and JNN Hospital
Kalyani, Dist. Nadia, West Bengal

PEEPEE
PUBLISHERS AND DISTRIBUTORS (P) LTD.

Pharmacology of Essential Medicines

Published by
Pawaninder P. Vij and Anupam Vij
Peepee Publishers and Distributors (P) Ltd.
Head Office: 160, Shakti Vihar, Pitam Pura
Delhi-110034 (India)

Correspondence Address: **7/31, First Floor, Ansari Road Daryaganj, New Delhi-110002 (India)**

Ph: 65195868, 23246245, 9811156083

e-mail: peepee160@yahoo.co.in

e-mail: peepee160@rediffmail.com

e-mail: peepee160@gmail.com

www.peepeepub.com

First Edition : 2015

ISBN: 978-81-8445-174-0

DEDICATED

TO

THE EXPERIMENTAL

ANIMALS

PREFACE

The common people, the common diseases are treated by "Essential drugs". There are many books in pharmacology, but drugs containing pharmacology of essential drugs are rare so far my knowledge goes. In this book, I have tried to compile pharmacology of the essential drugs. The essential drugs are available as generic drug name. Here some proprietory brand names are also given.

I thank my college seniors, Dr. B.R. Ghosh (Medical Superintendent of COMJNM Hospital, Prof. D. Bhattacharya (Principal, COM and JNMH), Dr. Bhaskar, Dr. Ritesh Singh or Prof. Kalyan Bhattacharya, Dr. (Mrs.) Susmita Bhattacharya, Dr. S. Roy, Dr. (Mrs.) Chitra Chatterjee, Prof. S. Deb (Ex. Principal, COMJNM Hospital), Dr. Utpal Biswas, Prof. B.L. Pandey (Dept. of Pharmacology, IMS, BHU), Dr. T. Deb, Dr. Kushal Banerjee and Dr. Chanchal Dalai, Dr. Abhisek Ghosh, my students Mr. A. Parveen, Mr. Abhinab, Mr. Chayan Manna, all who encouraged to write this book.

Mr. Pawaninder P. Vij, Director of Peepee Publishers and Distributors (P) Ltd. helped me to give my manuscript in this book form. My special thanks to them all.

K. MUKHOPADHYAY
Prof. and H.O.D.
Dept. of Pharmacology
College of Medicine and JNN Hospital
Kalyani, Dist. Nadia, West Bengal

CRITERIA FOR SELECTING ESSENTIAL DRUGS

- Its choice depends upon disease prevalence, available finance resources, genetic and demographic and environmental factors.
- When two drugs are available, choice is made on relative efficiency, safety, price, cost, benefits and pharmacokinetics studies.
- Generally it is a simple drug with few fixed drug combinations.
- Its selection is continuous process depending upon public health.
- Available safety data should be available from its clinical studies.
- It should be available in stable and storage form including bio-availability.

In this book WHO and Indian essential drug lists are discussed in details. The drugs are arranged alphabetically. Since essential medicine list is always changing in this look essential drugs of 2007 is covered.The essential medicine requirement of primary, secondary and tertiary health care are different.

CONTENTS

ABACAVIR (ABC)

It is included in WHO essential medicine list. It is guanosine analog, Nucleoside and Nucleotide reverse transcriptase inhibitors.

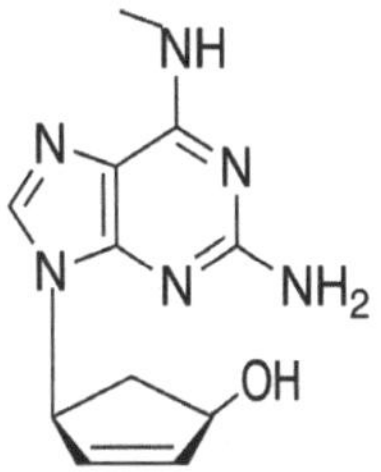

It is absorbed orally, food does not interfere absorption, CSF level is 1/3 of plasma.

ADR: Hypersensitivity (may be fatal), fever, malaise, nausea, vomiting, diarrhoea, anorexia, dyspnoea, pharyngitis, cough, skin rash may occur, serum amino transaminase, creatinine kinase, may increase pancreatitis. Alcohol should be avoided.

Available as 300 mg tab.

Dose: 300 mg BD or 600 mg OD.

Resistance develops slowly due to mutation. Cross resistance is also seen.

TRADE NAME : ABAVIR; ABAMUNE.

ACENOCOUMAROL

It is enlisted in Indian essential medicine list.

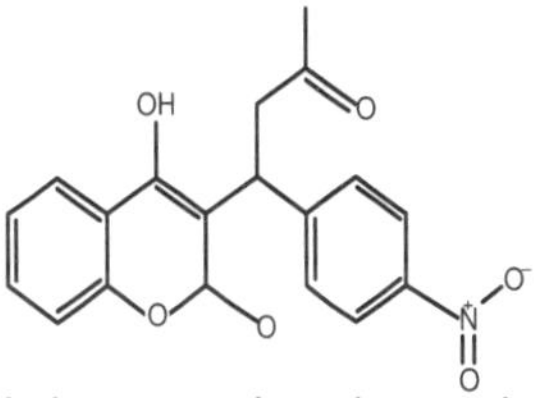

It is an oral anticoagulant. Its t/2 is 8 hours but its active metabolites make it 24 hours. It is available on 1, 2, 4 mg tablets.

ADR: Bleeding from different sites. Dose adjustment should be done measuring prothombine time.

Treatment of bleeding produced by it is:

(i) Stop the drug (ii) Vitamin K (iii) Fresh blood or frozen plasma.

TRADE NAME: ACITORM

ACETAZOLAMIDE

Enlisted in WHO and Indian essential medicine list.

This is a sulfonamide derivative, non competitive and reversibly inhibits carbonic anhydrase (CA). It acts as (i) Diuretics

(ii) Decreases intraocular tension (iii) Decreases gastric hydrochloric acid and pancreatic secretion (iv) Raises CO_2 level of brain and reduces pH of CSF and thereby increases seizure threshold (v) Alters CO_2 transport of lungs.

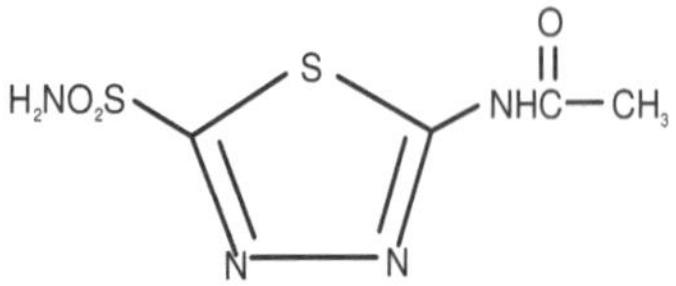

Orally absorbed and excreted with urine.

Uses: (i) Glaucoma (ii) Alkalinise urine (iii) Epilepsy as adjuvant (iv) Periodic paralysis (v) Acute mountain sickness.

Dose: 250 mg OD to BD.

Available as 250 tab.

ADR: Hypokalaemia, Acidosis, Drowsiness, Paraesthesia, Fatigue, Hypersensitivity, Bone marrow depression, Acidosis in COPD patient, Hepatic coma in liver disease may occur.

TRADE NAME : DIAMOX; SYNOMAX.

ACETYL CYSTEINE

Enlisted in WHO essential medicine list.

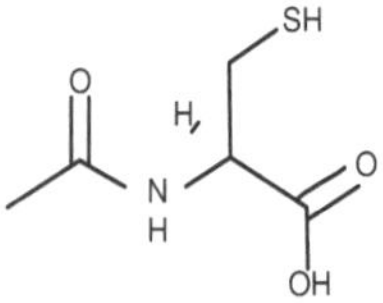

This mucolytic opens the disulfide bond present in the mucoproteins of sputum to decrease its viscocity.

It is directly administered in respiratory tract.

Available as 200 mg / ml inj. in 1, 2, 5 ml ampoules. It has to be nebulized or injected through tracheostomy tube.

TRADE NAME: MUCOMIX.

ACETYL – SALICYLIC ACID (ASPIRIN)

It is enlisted both in WHO and Indian essential medicine list.

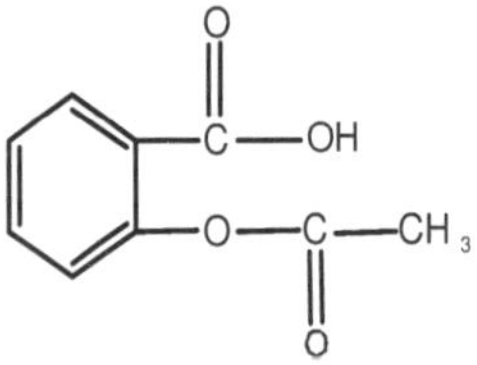

Converted in body to salicylic acid and other actions are due to acetylation of COX.

It is absorbed from stomach and intestine. It is deacetylated in gut wall, liver, plasma to release salicylic acid. It is protein bound 80%, enters brain and crosses placenta. It conjugates with glycine and glucuronic acid. Metabolites are excreted by filtration of kidney and secretion by tubule which can be enhanced by alkalinization

ADR: Nausea, vomiting, occult blood loss, rash, urticaria, rhinorrhea, angioedema, asthma, anaphylactoid reaction, dizziness, tinnitus, vertigo, hyperventilation, electrolyte imbalance, raises serum aminotransferase. Reye's syndrome, *salicylate poisoning* if taken above 15-30 gm presents with vomiting, dehydration acidosis, hypo or hyperglycaemia, petecheal haemorrhage, restlessness, hyperpyrexia, convulsion and coma.

The treatment of salicylate poisoning is symptomatic and supportive viz—Cooling, I.V. fluid administration, gastric lavage, forced alkaline diuresis, haemodialysis blood transfusion and Vitamin K.

It should not be given to patient with bleeding tendencies, liver diseases, children below 12 years and glucose 6- PO_4 deficient patient. It should be stopped before surgery and pregnancy.

Uses: Analgesic; Antipyretic; Acute rheumatic fever, Rheumatoid arthritis; Post stroke and infarction patient.

Available 350 mg tab, 75, 150, 325 mg tabs.

Interactions:

i. Being protein bound displaces warfarin, sulfonylurea, phenytoin, methotrexate.
ii. Inhibits secretion of uric acid by renal tubules.
iii. Blunts diuretic effect of frusemide and thiazides.

TRADE NAME: ASPIRIN; ECOSPRIN; DISPRIN.

ACRIFLAVIN + GLYCERIN

Included in essential medicine list of India.

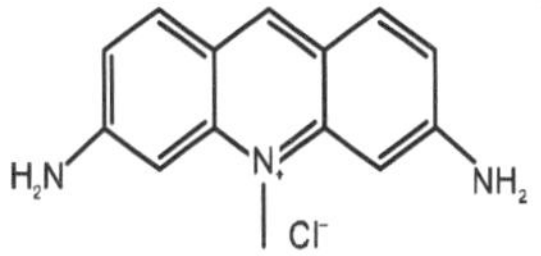

Acredine dye is yellow, orange, active against gram positive cocci and gonococci. Its efficacy is enhanced in alkaline medium. It looses efficacy on exposure to light, so kept in amber bottle. Applied over chronic ulcer, burn dressing. *Triple dye* contains gentian violet 0.25% + Brilliant green 0.25% + Acredine 0.1% applied over umbilical stump of newborn.

Glycerin: Clear, sweet and viscous liquid produces a warm sensation and irritates mucous membrane. Applied over dry skin, lips, vehicle for gum and throat paint.

When used orally per rectum (50-75%) or I.V. as (10%) reduces intraocular and intracranial pressure.

TRADE NAME: ACRINOL 0.1% cream.

ACTINOMYCIN–D (DACTINOMYCIN)

It is included in WHO and Indian essential medicine list.

It is obtained from *Streptomyces* organism. It inhibits DNA dependent RNA synthesis by binding double stranded DNA through intercalation between adjacent guanosine-cytosine base pairs.

Therapeutically used for pediatric tumors (Wilm's tumors, Rhabdomyosarcoma, Ewing sarcoma), Choriocarcinoma.

ADR: Nausea, Vomiting, Stomatitis, G.I. upset, Alopecia, Bone marrow depression may occur.

Available as 0.5 mg/vial.

Dose: 15 microgram/kg/I.V. × 5 days.

TRADE NAME: DACMOZEN.

ACTIVATED CHARCOAL

It is included in WHO and Indian essential medicine list.

It is prepared destructive distillation of vegetable matter (saw dust, cellulose, residue, coconut shells etc.) treated with zinc chloride to increase adsorptive power, the residue left is activated wood charcoal. It is black, odourless, tasteless powder free from grit.

Therapeutic Uses

i. Flatulence, dyspepsia, diarrhoea.
ii. In suspension with water for gastric lavage for emergency treatment of poisoning with alkaloids (morphine, strychnine, atropine).

It is a constituent of universal antidote given by mouth 4 to 8 gram (2 parts), other constituents are magnesium oxide (one part) and tannic acid (one part).

Charcoal can interfere with absorption of antibiotics.

Home Made Universal Antidote

Burn toast (2 parts).

Strong tea (1 part).

Milk of magnesia or chalk (1 part).

ACYCLOVIR

It is enlisted both in WHO and Indian essential medicine list.

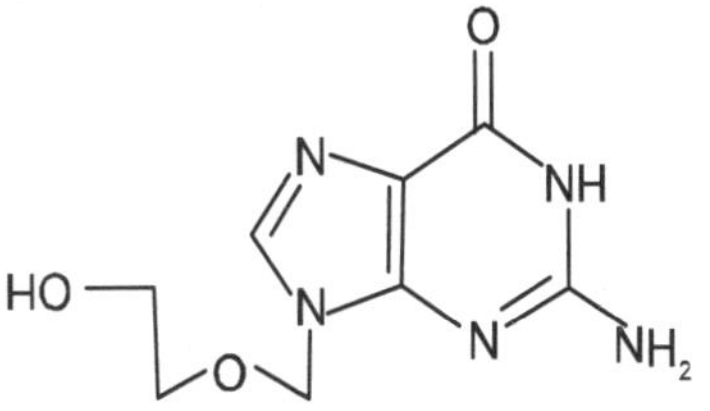

This antiviral agent is effective against HSV-1, HSV-2, VZV. In vitro its activity is noted against EBV, CMV and human herpes virus-6

This guanosine derivative antiviral agent undergoes three phosphorylation before activation.

First it is converted to monophosphate derivative by virus specific thymidine kinase and then to di and tri phosphate compounds by host cell enzymes. Acyclovir tri phosphate inhibits viral DNA synthesis.

It is orally absorbed, food does not interfere with its absorption. It may be topically used or be given I.V. It is little plasma protein bound, enters CSF, cornea. It is excreted with urine by filtration and secretion, so dose adjustment requires for kidney impaired patients.

Therapeutic Uses:

i. Genital herpes simplex (Dose 1 gm/Day × 10 days).
ii. Mucocutaneous herpes simplex (15 mg/kg/day × 7-8 days).
iii. Herpes simplex encephalitis 10-20 mg/kg/8 hourly I.V. × 10 days.
iv. Herpes simplex (type 1 keratitis).
v. Herpes zoster 10 mg/kg 8 hourly I.V. × 7 days or 800 mg orally 5 times a day.
vi. Chicken pox: 15 mg/kg/day I.V. × 7 days in immunodeficiency patient. Orally 400 mg QDS × 7 days may abort susceptible contacts.

Available as 200 mg tab, 250 mg/vial for I.V. 5% skin cream, 3% eye oint.

TRADE NAME: OCUVIR.

ADENOSINE

It is enlisted in Indian essential medicine list.

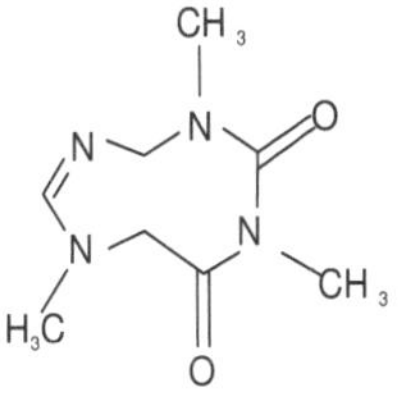

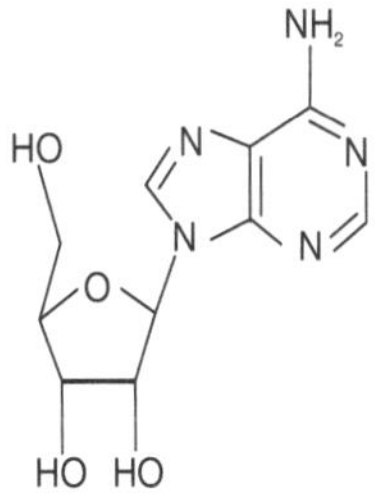

Adenosine is nucleoside present in body naturally. It activates inward rectifier K^+ current and inhibits Ca current causing hyperpolarization and suppression of calcium dependent action potential. Its t/2 is about 10 seconds because it is taken up by RBC and endothelial cells, where it is converted to 5 AMP and inosine.

Its action is potentiated by dipyridamole and blocked by theophylline.

It produces transient dyspnoea, chest pain, fall in BP, ventricular standstill, bronchospasm.

Therapeutic Uses:

i. PSVT.

ii. To diagnose tachycardia dependent on A.V. node.

iii. Brief coronary vasodilatation during diagnosis and interventions.

iv. Produce controlled hypotension.

Available as 3 mg adenosine base/ml in 2 ml and 10 ml ampoules.

TRADE NAME: ADENOCOR.

ALBENDAZOLE

Included in WHO and Indian essential medicine list.

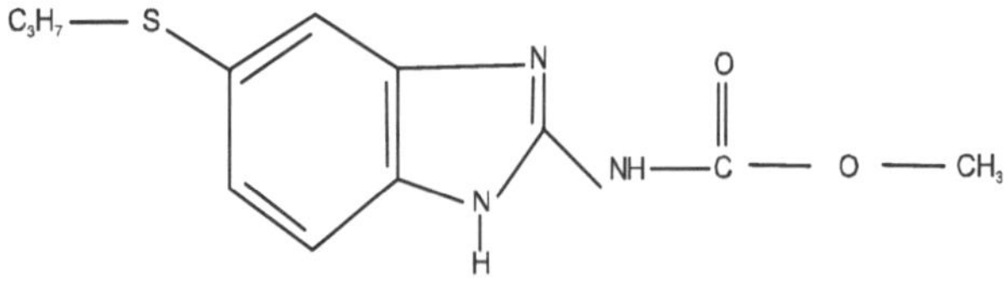

This congener of mebendazole has broad spectrum of action, against helminth, single dose oral administration. Chemically it is benzimidazole carbamate. When used for luminal parasite, it is given in empty stomach and for tissue parasite; it is given after fatty meal.

It is used for: Ascaris, Hookworm, Enterobius, Trichuris, Tapeworm, Strongyloidosis, Trichinosis, Neurocysticercosis.

Dose: 15 mg/kg/day × 15 days. Cutaneous larva migrans (400 mg × 3 days).

Hydatid disease (400 mg BD × 4 weeks). Filariasis as adjuvant to diethylcarbamazine.

It is well tolerated. G.I. upset, headache, fever, alopecia, jaundice, neutropenia may occur on prolong use. It is embryotoxic, so contraindicated in pregnancy.

Available as 400 mg tab, 200 mg/5 ml suspension.

TRADE NAME: ZENTAL.

ALBUMIN

Included in essential medicine list of India.

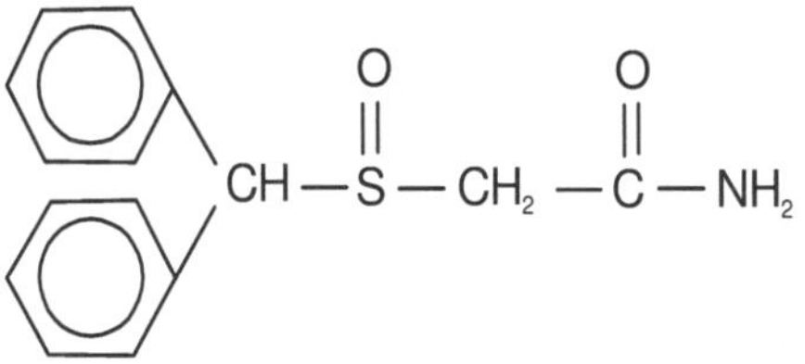

Human albumin is obtained from pooled human plasma. 100 ml of 20% human albumin solution is osmotically equivalent to 400 ml of frozen plasma or 800 ml of whole blood.

It can be given to any blood group without risk of transmitting hepatitis (because it is heat treated).

Crystalloid fluid should be used concurrently.

Therapeutic Uses:

i. Burn.
ii. Shock.
iii. Hypoproteinemia.
iv. Acute liver failure.
v. Dialysis.
vi. Dilution of blood with albumin and crystalloid before cardiopulmonary bypass.

It is expensive. Fever may occur.

Available as 20%.

TRADE NAME: ALBUDAC 50, 100 ml injection.

ALCURONIUM

Included in WHO's essential medicine list.

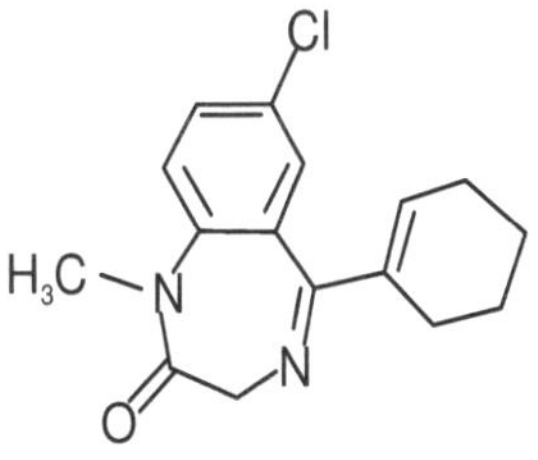

Alcuronium is non-depolarizing skeletal muscle relaxant obtained from *Chondrodendron tomentosum* and *Strychnos toxifera* with structural modification of C-toxiferine obtained from those plants alkaloid.

Its speed of onset duration of action etc. are like d-tubocurarine. but dose is less. It is reversed by anti-cholinergic agents. There is no apparent benefit over d-tubocurarine.

ALLOPURINOL

Enlisted in WHO and Indian essential medicine list.

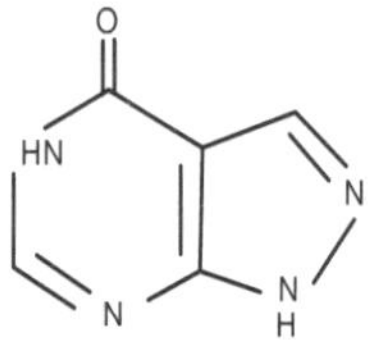

Allopurinol is xanthine oxidase inhibitor and thereby reduces uric acid level and so used for gouty arthritis.

It is 80% absorbed after oral absorption. It is itself metabolized by xanthine oxidase to produce alloxanthine which also have got xanthine oxidase inhibiting capacity, so it is long acting given once daily. Colchicine should be simultaneously used, till uric acid level goes to 6 mg/dl.

ADR: G.I. intolerance, nausea, vomiting, diarrhea, peripheral neuritis, necrotizing vasculitis, bone marrow depression, hepatic toxicity, nephritis, allergic skin lesion, exfoliative dermatitis etc. have been reported.

Dose: 100 mg/day.

Liberal fluid should be permitted.

Therapeutic Uses:

i. Chronic gout.
ii. Secondary gout of cancer chemotherapy, radiation and diuretics.
iii. To potentiate 6-mercaptopurine or azathioprine or immuno-suppressant therapy.

Available as 100 and 300 mg tabs.

Dose: 100 mg OD to 300 μg /day.

TRADE NAME: ZYLORIC .

ALFA - INTERFERON

It is enlisted in essential medicine list of India.

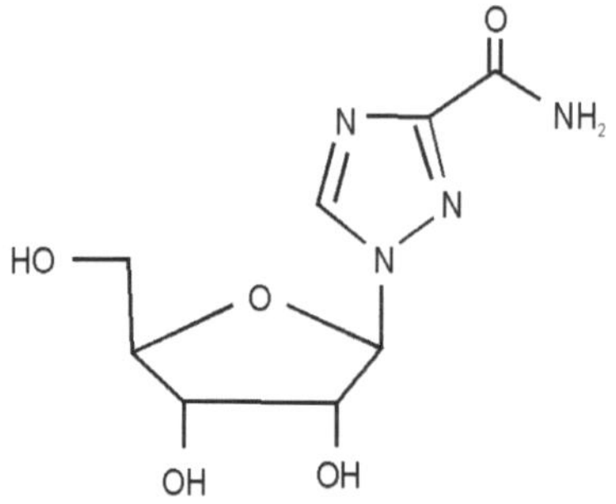

Interferons are produced by host cells in response to viral infection. These are low molecular weight glycoprotein cytokines. It has non-specific antiviral as well as other effects on immunity and cell proliferation. It binds to receptor of cell surface and affects viral replication. Its receptor is JAK-STAT tyrosine protein kinase. Interfereon inhibits RNA and DNA virus and are host specific.

Interferon α, β and γ have been produced by recombinant DNA technology. Interfereon α_{2A} and α_{2B} have antiviral activity. It is given I.M. or I.V. Interfereon α_{2A} is available as ALFERON 3 MU/vial.

It is used for:

i. Chronic hepatitis by B and C virus.
ii. AIDS related Kaposi's sarcoma.
iii. Immunocompromised host with HSV, HZV and CMV infection.
iv. Intranasal interferon for rhinovirus.
v. It is also used for CML and multiple myeloma.

ADR: Flu like feature, visual disturbance, myelosuppression, neurotoxicity, hypotension, alopecia, arrhythmia, liver dysfunction, hypo or hyperthyroidism may occur.

ALPRAZOLAM

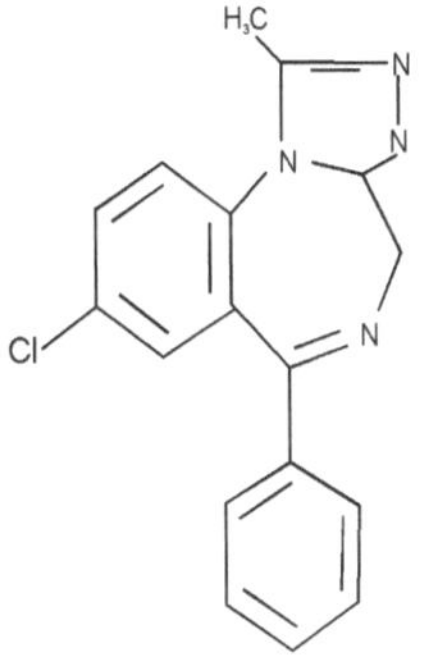

Alprozolam is anxiolytic benzodiazepines which has also mood elevating properties, particularly useful when anxiety is markedly co-existing with depression. It is also effective for panic.

It is orally effective. It undergoes α-hydroxylation, the metabolites produced; produces short lived pharmacological effect because it rapidly conjugates with glucuronides which is inactive and excreted with urine. Discontinuation after regular use produces withdrawl phenomenon.

Hypnotic dose 0.25 to 0.5 mg.

Dose: 0.25 to 1 mg TDS upto 6 mg/day for panicky patient.

Available as 0.25, 0.5, 1mg tab 1.5 mg SR tab.

COMMON TRADE NAME: ALZOLAM.

ALUMINIUM ACETATE

It is included in WHO essential medicine list.

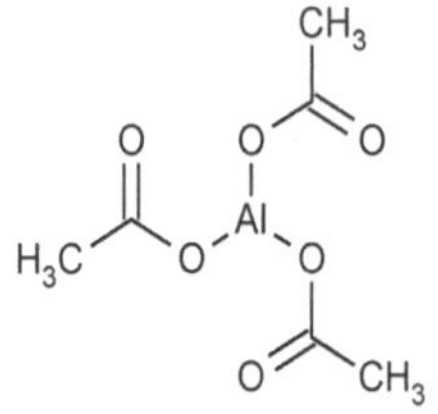

Marketed as Burrow's solution and is used to treat external ear disease. Burrow's solution has anti-inflammatory, anti-pruritic, astringent properties. It does not sensitize skin, well tolerated and does not produce resistance organism. It is used to irrigate ear and to remove debris.

ALUMINIUM HYDROXIDE + MAGNESIUM HYDROXIDE

It is enlisted in Indian essential medicine list.

Used as antacid combination to treat peptic ulcer. The benefit of combinations are as following:

i. Magnesium hydroxide is fast acting but aluminium hydroxide is slow acting.
ii. Magnesium hydroxide is laxative but aluminium hydroxide is constipating.
iii. Dose of individual component is reduced, so the side effects.

Antacids are generally self-administered. It is used for non ulcer dyspepsia, heart burn and GERD.

AMIKACIN

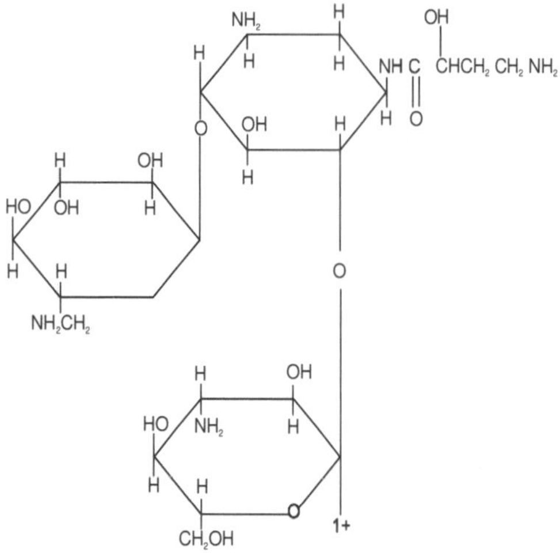

It is water soluble semisynthetic derivative of kanamycin obtained from acylation. It is not inactivated by bacterial aminoglycoside inactivating enzyme. Susceptible organisms are *E. coli, Klebsiella* pneumoniae, *Pseudomonas* aeruginosa, serratia, providencia, *Enterobacter, Staph aureus* and *albus* are also sensitive but should not be used for these gram positive organisms, because safe antibiotics are available for those. It is also effective for *M. tuberculosis*, but rarely used. Shares all the properties and toxicities of aminoglycosides (hearing loss is more than vestibular disturbance).

Dose: 15 mg/kg/day in 2-3 divided doses, for U.T.I. dose is 7.5 mg/kg/day given I.M. or I.V.

Available as 150 mg, 250 mg, 500 mg/2 ml injection.

Precaution: Serum amikacin and creatinine level should be assessed periodically.

TRADE NAME: AMICIN; MICACIN.

AMILORIDE

It is included in WHO essential medicine list.

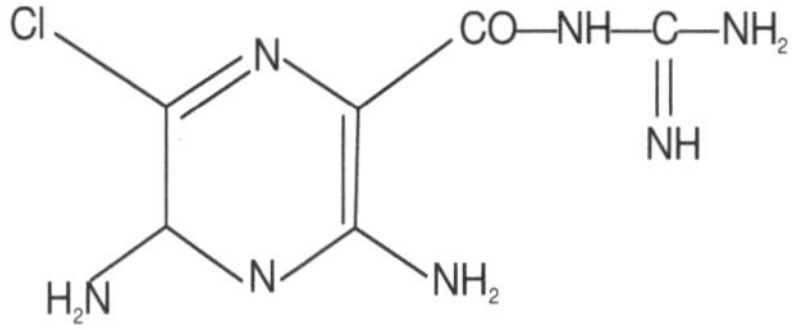

This potassium sparing diuretic is direct inhibitor of Na^+ influx in collecting tubule. It is non-steroidal organic base.

It is used with thiazide or high ceiling diuretic to prevent K sparing. Concurrent K supplementation may produce dangerous hyperkalaemia. ß blockers and ACE inhibitors are also likely to produce hyperkalaemia.

Dose: 5 mg.

Generally available as combination preparation.

AMINOPHYLLINE

It is included in Indian essential medicine list. Chemically it is theophylline ethylenediamine.

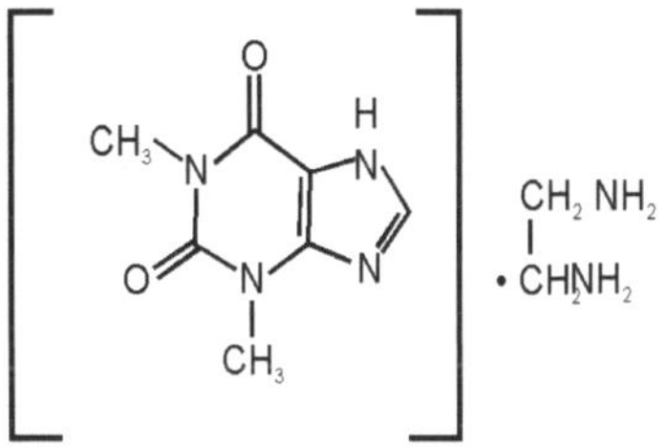

When given by slow intravenous injection it relieves acute bronchospasm or status asthmaticus that is resistant to adrenergic drugs.

It inbibits phosphodiesterase inhibitors (PDE_4). It can be given orally, intramuscular or rectally. Intramuscular route is not preferred because it may produce prolong and severe pain. Oral route causes G.I. irritation and absorption is erratic.

Headache, dizziness, nervousness, nausea, vomiting, severe gastric pain may occur with oral administration. Prolonged use as suppositories causes rectal irritation, convulsion and shock. Rapid I.V. administration causes arrhythmia, profound hypotension, cardiac arrest. Persistent vomiting, agitation and convulsion may occur by any route. It is dangerous if cough preparations with theophylline and aminophylline are given concomitantly.

Dose: 250 mg in 10-20 ml of diluents injected cautiously over 5-10 minutes. If continuous infusion is required dose is 5-6 mg/kg over 30 minutes followed by 1 mg/kg/hr.

Dose for children 15 mg/kg/day in these divided doses. Loading dose 7mg/kg followed by 6-10 mg/kg/24 hours.

Available as 100 mg tab, 250 mg/10 ml injection.

P-AMINOSALICYLIC ACID (PAS)

It is included in WHO essential medicine list.

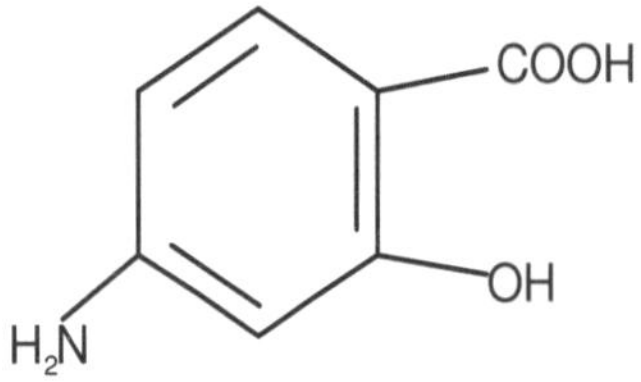

It was introduced in 1946, its mechanism of action is similar is sulfonamide. It is tuberculostatic. Until ethambutol was available. It was widely used combined chemotherapy of tuberculosis.

It is completely absorbed orally, and distributed widely except in CSF. It is acetylated. Some are slow and some are fast acelylator and it competes within acetylation for INH. Acceptibility of PAS is poor.

ADR: Nausea, anorexia, epigastric pain, rash, fever, goitre, liver dysfunction, blood dyscrasia.

Dose: 10-12 g/day or 200 mg/kg.

Available as 0.5 gm tab, 80 gm/100 gram granules.
TRADE NAME: SODIUM PAS.

AMIODARONE

Enlisted in essential medicine list of India.

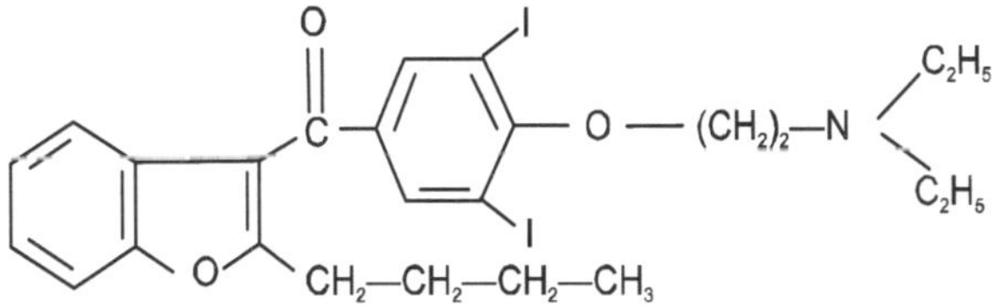

Amiodarone is used orally and I.V. for treating serious ventricular and supraventricular arrhythmia. It belongs to class III antiarrhythmic agent. It prolongs APD and QT interval due to myocardial delayed rectifier K^+ channel and preferentially block NA^+ channel. In spite of prolonging Ca^{2+} channel, its potentialities to produce torsades de pointes is low.

It is incompletely and slowly absorbed from GIT, administration on I.V. action starts quickly. It accumulates in muscle and fats and released slowly from there.

It is metabolized in liver, one of its metabolite is active.

Dose: Low dose of amiodarone (100-200 mg/day) effective for normal sinus rhythm after atrial fibrillation (AF). Dose per se is 400-600 mg/day followed by 100-200 mg OD or 5 mg/kg I.V. slowly over 30-60 minutes.

ADR: Hypotension, Bradycardia, nausea, G.I. upset, photosensitization, skin pigmentation, corneal microdeposit, pulmonary alveolities. Interferes with thyroid function and inhibits peripheral conversion of T_4 to T_3.

Interaction:

i. Increases digoxin and warfarin level by decreasing their renal clearance.
ii. A.V. block may increase if used with ß-blocker or calcium channel blocker.

Dose: 100 mg, 200 mg tab, 150 mg/3 ml injection.
TRADE NAME: CORDARONE.

AMITRIPTYLIN

Included in WHO and Indian essential medicine list.

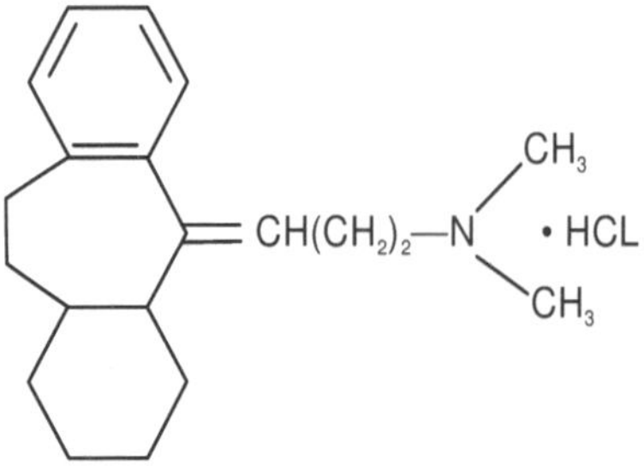

It is as effective as imipramine in the treatment of depression. Confusional episodes (more in elderly), weight gain, leucopenia may occur. It may produce sedation, dry mouth (antimuscarinic effect) hypotension, cardiac arrhythmia.

Available as 10, 25, 75 mg tab., 10 mg/ml in 10 ml containers.

Dose: I.M. 80-100 mg daily in four divided doses.

Adults (Hospitalized)100 mg/daily in divided doses or 10 mg TDS for adults elderly or 75 mg in three divided doses in outpatient patients. Other use aneurosis 25 mg at bed time.

TRADE NAME: TRYPTOMER; SEROTENA.

AMLODIPINE

Included in WHO and Indian essential medicine lists.

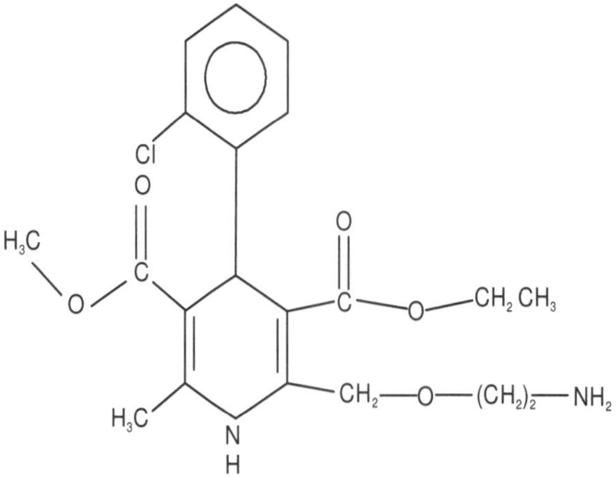

This is dihydropyridine (DHD) group of calcium channel blocker. It is completely and slowly absorbed form G.I.T. Palpitation, flushing, headache, dizziness, ankle oedema may occur. It is long acting.

Available in 2.5 mg, 5 mg and 10 mg tablets.

Dose: 5-10 mg OD.

S (-) enantiomer is effective in half doses and less likely to produce ankle oedema.

Therapeutic Uses: Hypertension, Angina.

S(-)enantiomer is marketed as S-Numlo 2.5, 5 mg tablets.

TRADE NAME: AMLOPIN; AMLOSAFE.

AMODIAQUINE

It is included in WHO essential medicine list.

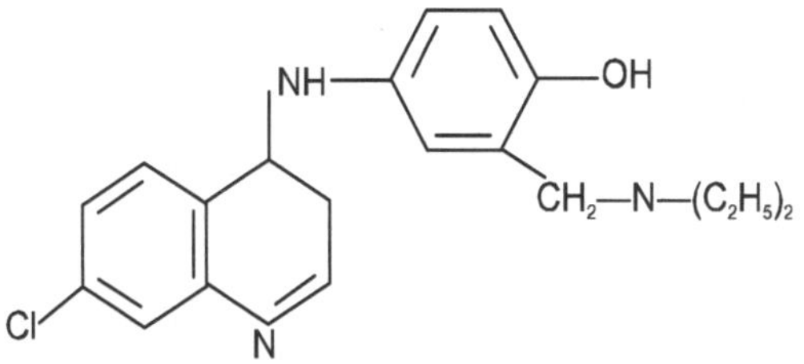

It is 4-aminoquinoline derivative. It is similar in action, mechanism of resistance that occur with chloroquine. It is cheap, low toxicity and effective in some chloroquine resistant *P. falciparum* patient.

ADR: G.I. intolerance, headache, photosensitivity, toxic hepatitis, agranulocytosis. It is not recommended for prophylaxis.

Available as 250 mg of salt (150 mg as base).

Dose: 25-35 mg/kg for 3 days.

TRADE NAME: CAMOQUIN.

AMOXICILLIN

This drug is enlisted in essential medicine list of WHO and India.

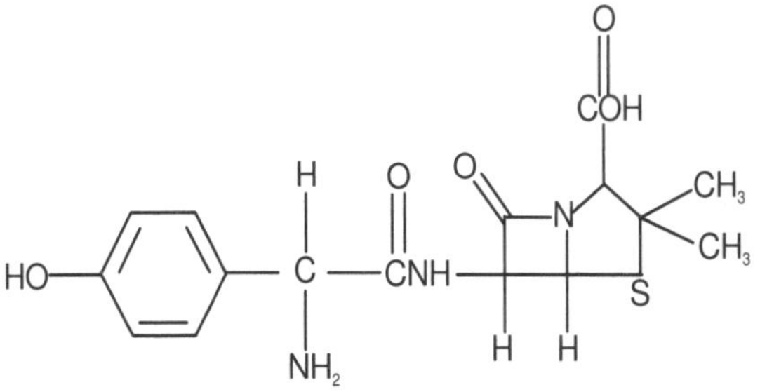

It is a semi-synthetic penicillin (Aminopenicillin) used orally and food does not interfere with its absorption. The incidence of diarrhea is less compared to ampicillin.

It is indicated to treat skin, soft tissue and lower respiratory tract infection by susceptible bacteria (Non-penicillinase producing).

It appears to be well-tolerated.

ADR: are nausea, vomiting, diarrhoea, hypersensitivity, rash, fever, anaemia, serum sickness like response, life threatening anaphylaxis reaction may occur, SGOT may rise, superinfections with *Enterobacter, Pseudomonas, Candida* may occur.

Dose: 0.25-1g TDS oral/I.M., Children 25-50 mg/kg/day.

Available as 125 mg/5 ml dry syrp, 250, 500 mg cap.
TRADE NAME: NOVAMOX; MOX.

AMOXICILLIN + CLAVULANIC ACID

Listed in WHO essential medicine list.

Clauvulanic acid obtained from *Streptomyces clavuligerus.* It inhibits wide varieties of class II to class V beta lactamase produced by gram positive and gram negative bacteria. It is called 'suicide inhibitor' because it is inactive after binding the enzyme. It is orally absorbed and its tissue distribution matches with amoxycillin and eliminated by glomerular filtration, but it is unaffected by probenecid. By its addition its activity is re-established with ß lactamase producing *S. aureus, N. gonorrhea, E. coli, Proteus, Klebsiella, Salmonella, Shigella.*

This combination is available as 250 mg Amoxicillin + 125 mg Clavulanic acid as tab, 500 mg Amoxicillin + 125 mg Clavulanic acid tab, Amoxicillin 1g + Clavulanic acid 0.2 gm vial for I.M. OR I.V.

ADR: G.I. tolerance poorer Stomatitis and Vaginitis with Candida, rash, hepatic injury may occur.

This Combination is Indicated for:

i. Skin and soft tissue infection.
ii. Intra-abdominal infection.
iii. Gynaecological infection.
iv. R.T.I.
v. Biliary infection.
vi. U.T.I.
vii. Gonorrhea.

TRADE NAME: AUGMENTIN.

AMPHOTERICIN – B

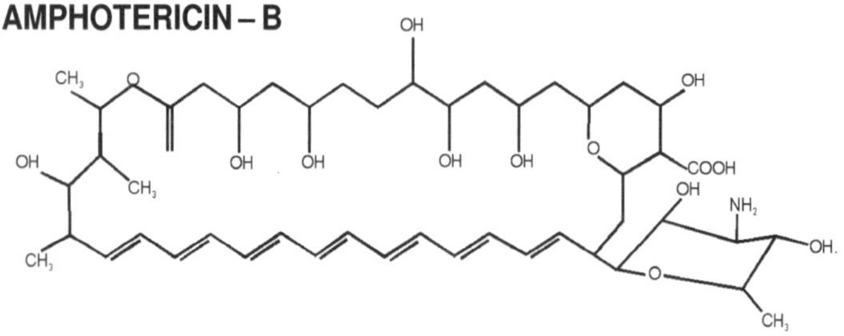

This antifungal antibiotic is included in essential medicine list of India and WHO, obtained from *Streptomyces nodosus.* It contains many double bonds polyene and a large lactone ring of 12 or more atoms (polyene macrolide). It is insoluble in water, so colloidal suspension of amphotericin B and desoxycholate are prepared for intravenous injection. It is poorly absorbed from G.I.T. I.V. drug administered is protein bound, metabolized and partly excreted with urine.

It has high affinity for ergosterol, present in fungal cell membrane and combines with it, to form microspores through which ions, amino acids and water soluble substances leak out.

Therapeutic Use:

i. Antifungal (*Candida, Histoplasma, Cryptococcus, Blastomyces, Coccidioides, Torulopsis*, Rhodotorula, Aspergillus, Sporothrix.

ii. *Leishmania.*

ADR: (A) Acute (Infusion related): Nausea, fever, ache, chill, vomiting, dyspnoea.

(B) Long term (cumulative): Nephrotoxicity, Anaemia.

(C) CNS toxicity (If given intrathecal): Headache, vomiting.

Dose (Oral): 50-100 mg QDS for intestinal monaliasis, 3% Ear drop (Fungizone otic) for otomycosis.

For systemic fungal infection I.V. dose 0.5 -1 mg/kg/day upto 1-2 g (Fungizone 50 mg/vial).

Newer Amphotericin B Formulations

(a) Amphotericin B lipid complex (ABLC).
(b) Amphotericin B colloidal dispersion (ABCD).
(c) Liposomal Amphotericin B.

Drug Interaction: Rifampicin, Minocycline potentiate, Amphotericin B, Flucytosine has supra additive action.

AMPICILLIN

Enlisted both in WHO and Indian essential medicine list.

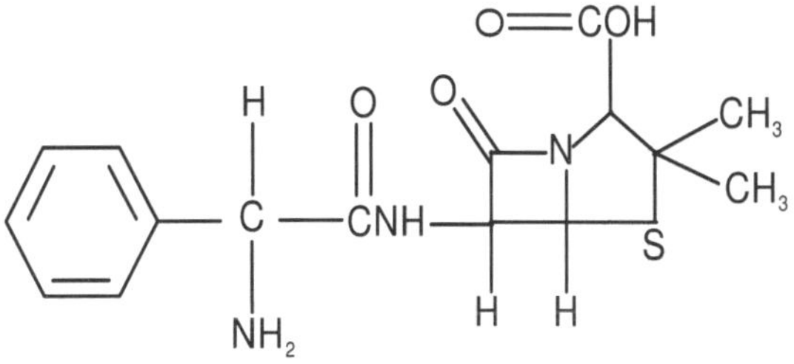

Apart of the organism effective by PNG it is effective against *H-influenzae, E-coli, Proteus, Salmonella, Shigella, Strep. viridans, Pneumo, Meningo and Gonococci* orally absorbed, food interferes absorption, partly excreted with bile (enterohepatic circulation) and by tubular secretion in kidney.

Therapeutic Uses: UTI, RTI, Meningitis, Gonorrhoea, Typhoid, Bacillary dysentry, Cholecystitis, Sub-acute bacterial endocarditis, Septicemia.

ADR: Rash (in AIDS, EB virus and lymphatic leukemia patient), Diarrhoea.

Interaction:

i. Hydrocortisone inactivates ampicillin if mixed in I.V.

ii. OCP may fail.

iii. Probenacid retards renal excretion.

Dose: 0.5-2 gm oral, I.M./I.V. per day.

Children 25-50 mg/kg/day.

Available as 250, 500 mg cap, 125 mg/5 ml dry syrup, 100 ml/ml drops, 250, 500; 1g/vial injection.

TRADE NAME : AMPILIN; ROSCILLIN etc.

ANTI-SNAKE VENOM SERUM

It is included in WHO and Indian essential medicine list.

It is purified, enzyme refined equine globulins in lyophilized vial supplied with 10 ml ampoules for reconstitution. Each ml can neutralize.

0.6 mg of cobra venom; 0.6 mg of Russel's viper venom.

0.45 mg of saw–sealed viper.

0.45 mg of krait.

It is given I.V. after negative skin testing. 20 ml I.V. (1ml /min) repeated every 6 hours till symptoms disappear, upto 300 ml. Higher does may be given (upto 600 ml) for cobra bite. Some serum is given around bite site in viper bite.

ADR: Allergy, Anaphylaxis.

Adrenaline should be kept at hand and given subcutaneous if reaction occurs.

TRADE NAME: ANTI-SNAKE VENOM SERUM POLYVALENT.

ANTI-D IMMUNO-GLOBULIN (HUMAN)

It is enlisted both in WHO and Indian essential medicine list.

It is IgG immunoglobulin with high titre of anibodies against Rh-D. It combines with RhO antigen and does not allow inducing antibody formation in Rh negative individual.

Therapeutic Uses:

1. Prevention of antibody formation in Rh negative mother delivered or aborted an Rh positive baby. Dose 250-350 microgram I.M.
2. Rh negative patient inadvertently administered Rh positive blood. Dose 1000-2000 microgram I.M.

TRADE NAME: RHIGGAL 100 - 350 microgram/vial.

ANTI-TETANUS IMMUNOGLOBIN (HUMAN)

Immunoglobulins are separated human globulins which carry the specific (hyper immune) antibodies against particular antigen which are more efficacious than antisera. Immunoglobulin tetanus (human) are indicated for prophylaxis in non-immunized person with a contaminated wound who is at risk of developing tetanus. It maintains a significant blood level for upto 14 weeks. If tetanus toxoid is given to the same individual but at different sites the primary immune response of the same is not interfered. It has also been tried intrathecally.

Dose: Prophylactic 250-500 I.U.
Therapeutic 3000-6000 I.U.] Given intramuscular

TRADE NAME: TETNAL 250 I.U./2 ml inj.

ARTEMETHER

It is included in WHO essential medicine list.

Artemether is prodrug. It is obtained from Chinese traditional plant Quinghasu, Artemisia annua the active principle of the plant is Artemisinis. Several derivatives of it are found, artemether is one of them. It is lipid soluble, administered orally or I.M. It undergoes first pass metabolism and is converted to dihydroartemisinin

Available as 40 mg cap, 80 mg/ml of arachis oil.

Therapeutic Use:

1. Used for uncomplicated/Chloroquine/multi-drug resistant falciparum malaria (used orally).
2. Severe and complicated falciparum malaria.

Drug Interaction: Simultaneous use of arteminisinin and terfenadine/Astemizole/Tricyclic anti-depressants may produce cardiac conduction defects.

TRADE NAME: METHILEX

ARTEMETHER + LUMEFANTRINE (1:6 ratio)

This fixed drug combination is enlisted in WHO's essential medicine list.

Lumefantrine is orally active, highly effective, long acting erythrocytic malarial schizontocide. It is used only in combination with artemether. Combination prevents development of resistance. It is administered with food, preferably fatty meal or milk to enhance their absorption.

ADR: Headache, Dizziness, Sleep disturbances, Abdominal pain, Arthralgia, Pruritis, Rash.

Drug Interactions: With Metoprolol, Neuroleptics, Tricyclic antidepressants may occur.

Dose: Artemether 80 mg BD.

Lumefantrine 480 mg BD.

TRADE NAME: COARTEM, LUMERAX.

ARTISUNATE

This artemisinin compound is included in the essential medicine list of both WHO and India.

Its sodium salt is water soluble and can be administered oral, I.M or I.V. Its oral absorption is fast but incomplete. Rapidly converted to active metabolite dihydroartemisinin.

Available as 50 mg tab, 60 mg/vial injection.

Used for:

1. Uncomplicated resistant falciparum malaria.
2. Severe and complicated falciparum malaria.

Dose: 4 mg/kg/day × 3 days.

Or 100 mg BD × 3 days.

TRADE NAME: FALCIGO.

ASCORBIC ACID (Vitamin C)

It is included both in WHO and Indian essential medicine list.

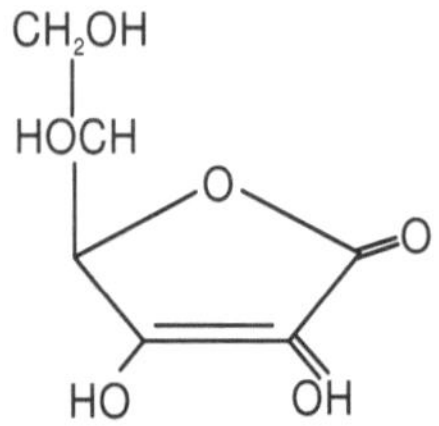

It is essential co-enzyme for collagen formation, tissue repair and synthesis of lipid and protein. It acts both as reducing agent and as an antioxidant which is necessary for many physiological functions (metabolism of iron, folic acid, resistance to infection and preservation of blood vessels integrity).

Dietary Source: Fresh fruits, vegetables, amla citrous fruits, linen. It is readily absorbed and after tissue saturation. Deficiency produces scurvy.

Therapeutic Uses: Vit C deficiency, Scurvy, Post operatively, Anaemia, to acidify urine, large doses are tried for common cold, cancer etc but results are inconsistent.

Mega doses for long period may produce rebound scurvy.

Available as 500 mg tabs, 100 mg/ml oral drops.

50 mg/2 ml for I.M.

Intramuscular preparation Cevalin.

TRADE NAME: Tab and Drops: CECON.

ATENOLOL

Included in WHO and Indian essential medicine list.

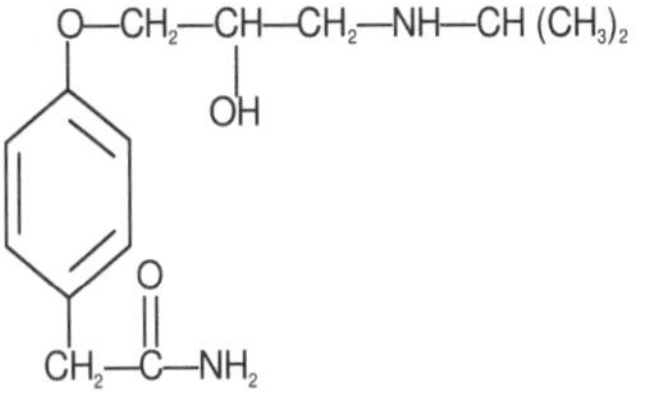

It is second generation β_1 selective, i.e., cardio selective β–adrenergic blocking drug. It is low lipid soluble. Incompletely absorbed from oral route taken once daily because of long action. Lipid profile not much affected.

Therapeutic Uses:

i. Hypertension.

ii. Angina.

Dose: 25-100 mg/day.

Available as 25, 50, 100 mg tab.

For S(-) Atenolol enantiomer, dose in half.

The side effects and contraindications of beta blockers should be kept in mind, before prescribing.

TRADE NAME: ATEN; BETACARD.

ATRACURIUM

It is included in Indian essential medicine list.

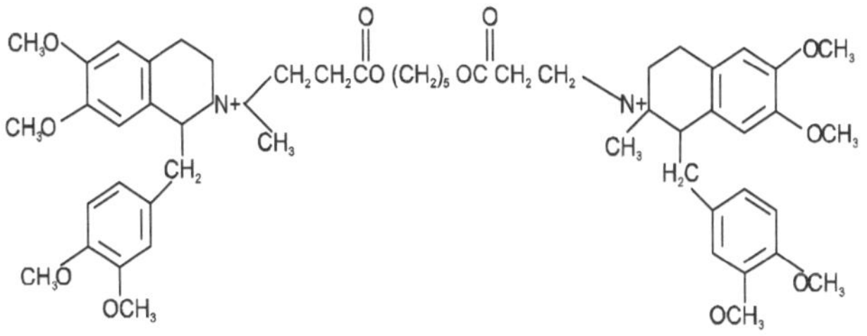

Atracurium is non-depolarizing neuro-muscular relaxants. It is short acting, reversal not required. It is inactivated by spontaneous non-enzymatic degradation called Hofman's elimination and in addition by cholinesterase, so its duration is not altered by hepatic and kidney insufficiency. It is preferred as muscle relaxant in neonates, elderly and in hepatic and renal insufficient patient. It releases histamine, so may produce hypotension.

Available as 10 mg / ml in 2ml vial.

TRADE NAME: TRACRIUM.

ATROPINE

Enlisted both in WHO and Indian national essential medicine list.

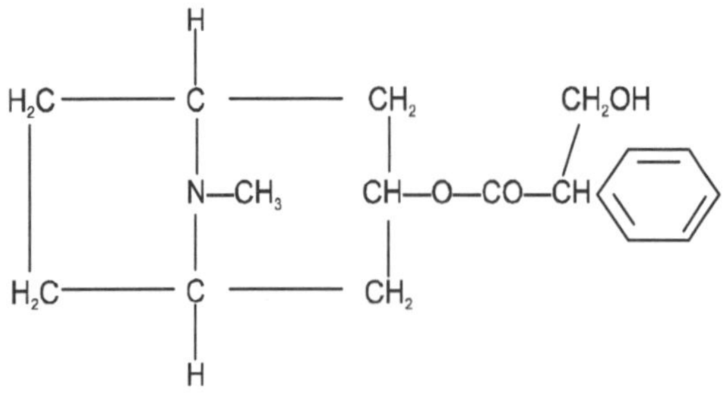

Atropine is an ester of an organic tropic acid with organic base tropine. It is one of the alkaloids of *Atropa belladona.* Atropine is (dl) hyoscyamin.

Therapeutic Uses:

i. As antispasmodic.
ii. Peptic ulcer.
iii. Eye for mydriasis and cycloplegia.
iv. Preanaesthetic medication.
v. Organophosphorous poisoning.
vi. Parkinsonism.
vii. A.V. block.

Precautions for Atropine Therapy

i. Patient over 40 years.
ii. Enlarged prostrate.
iii. CCF with tachycardia.
iv. Pyloric obstruction.

Available as:

i. Atropine sulfate 0.6 mg tabs. Dose 0.25 to 2 mg.
ii. Atropine eye ointment 1% in standard ointment base.
iii. Atropine sulfate injection 0.5 mg/ml ampoules.

AZATHIOPRINE

Included in WHO and Indian national essential medicine list.

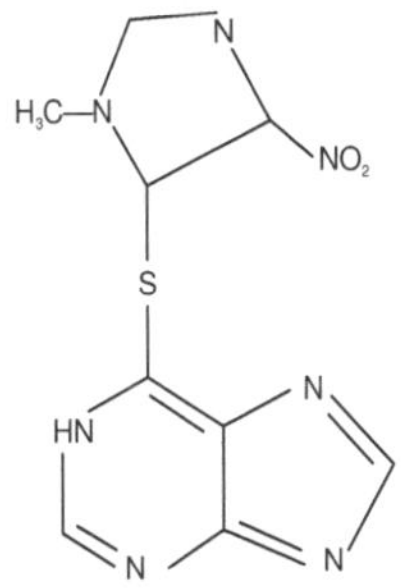

This drug is purine antagonist has marked effect on T-lymphocytes. It suppresses the cell mediated immunity, so apart from its action as anti-cancer drug it is used for organ transplantation, rheumatoid arthritis.

It is orally incompletely absorbed, metabolized by xanthine oxidase (so inhibited by xanthine oxidase inhibitors allopurinol).

Main toxic effects of azathioprine are bone narrow suppression, hyperuricaemia.

Dose: 3-5 mg/kg/day. Maintenance 1-2 mg/kg /day.

Available as 50 mg tab.

TRADE NAME: IMURAN.

AZITHROMYCIN

It is included in Indian and WHO essential medicine list.

It is azalide congener of erythromycin. More active against *H. influenzae* than other macrolides. It is effective against *Mycoplasma, Chlamydia, Legionella, Moraxella, Campylobactor, H ducreyi, N. gonorrhoea and MAC, Donovanosis.*

It is rapidly orally absorbed, acid stable with better tissue distribution and penetration. Once daily dosing.

Used for pharyngitis, tonsillitis, sinusitis, otitis media, pneumonia, chronic bronchitis, skin and soft tissue infection, MAC in AIDS, typhoid, toxoplasmosis, malaria.

Available as 250, 500 mg cap 250 mg/ml dry syrup.

ADR: G.I. upset, abdominal pain, headache, dizziness.

Less likely to produce interaction with theophylline, carbamazepine, warfarin, terfenadine.

TRADE NAME: AZITHRAL.

B.C.G. VACCINE

This is included in WHO and national essential medicine list of India.

It is live vaccine containing attenuated bovine strain of *M. tuberculosis* bacteria. Calmette and Guerin of France developed it in 1921. It is 0.5 -1mg of dry powder (1 - 2.5 $\times 10^7$ colony forming units in ampoules with 1ml of sterile water.

Dose: 0.05 ml for neonates and 0.1ml for older patients to be given intracutaneously in deltoid muscle at birth. In adults it is given only if tuberculine test is negative.

After giving it a painless papule appears after one week with swelling of axillary lymph node which may ulcerate and dries up in 3 months.

BCC vaccine also stimulates immunity and so also used as adjuvant of cancer. It should not be given to tuberculine positive, HIV positive and pregnant mothers.

BECLOMETHASONE DIPROPIONATE

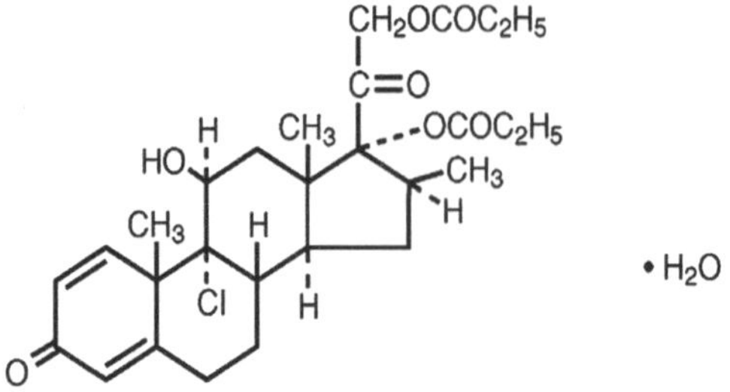

Beclomethasone dipropionate is a glucocorticoids with high topical and low systemic active steroid. It is available on 50,100, 200 mirogram/ metered dose inhaler. 100, 200, 400 microgram per cap with rotahaler.

It is also available as potent topical steroid. Beclomethasone dipropionate 0.025% cream.

The inhaler is used for bronchial asthma. The topical steroid is used for atopic eczema; allergic contact dermatitis, lichen simplex, dermatitis, seborrheic dermatitis, psoriasis, varicose eczema, cystic acne, alopecia areata, DLE, keloid, hypertrophied scars, lichen planus.

BENZATHINE BENZYLPENICILLN

Included in WHO and Indian essential medicine list.

Per se penicillin is narrow spectrum antibiotic. Benzathine penicillin is long acting. Available as 0.6, 1.2, 2.4 MU of the drug given deep I.M. every 2-4 weeks.

It is like other benzyl penicillin used for:

i. *Streptococcal.*
ii. *Pneumococcal.*
iii. *Meningococcal.*
iv. *Gonococcal.*
v. *Syphilis.*
vi. *Diphtheria.*
vii. *Tetanus.*
viii. *Gas gangrene.*
ix. *Trench mouth.*
x. *Listeria monocytogenes.*

Prophylactically for: Rheumatic fever, Bacterial endocarditis, Agranulocytosis patient.

ADR: It is generally non-toxic. Local irritancy at injection site, hypersensitivity, superinfection, Jarisch-Herxheimer reaction may occur.

It is advisable to inject Benzathine benzyl penicillin only if it is giving negative skin testing.

BENZOIC ACID + SALICYLIC ACID

This combination preparation used topically. It is included in WHO and Indian essential medicine list.

Benzoic acid has anti-fungal and anti-bacterial property.

Salicylic acid as 10-20% solution in alcohol or propylene glycol dissolves corns, if applied under occlusive dressing. It is keratolytic (i.e., dissolves intracellular substance in horny layer of skin). In lower concentration in combination with benzoic acid (benzoic acid 5% of salicylic acid 3% called whitfield ointment used in hyperkerotic lesion.

It may cause irritation and burning sensation.

BENZOIN COMPOUND

It is included in essential medicine list of India.

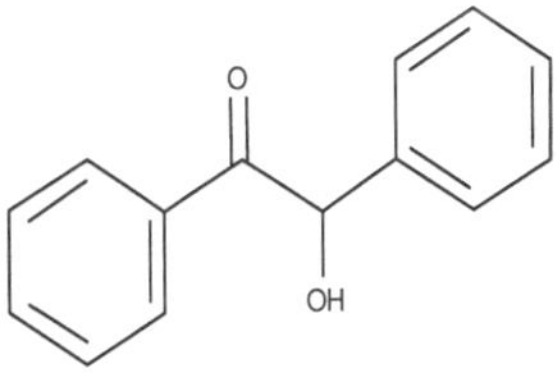

It is used as protective adhesive paint for cuts and abrasion on skin (Tincture benzoin co I.P.).

It is prepared as following:

Treatment:

Benzoin crushed	10 gm
Prepared storax	7.5 gm

Balsam of tolu	2.5 gm
Aloe	2.0 gm
Alcohol 90%	100 ml
M. Ft. solution	

Benzoin, storax and tolu are resins. Resins and aloe act as adhesive and protective. Alcohol acts as vehicle and antiseptic.

BENZOYL PEROXIDE

Included in WHO essential medicine list.

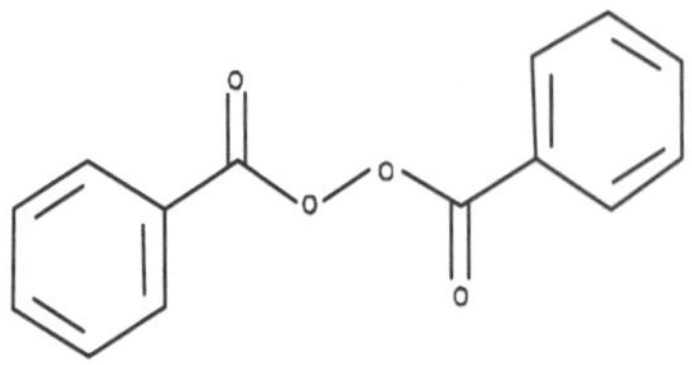

It gradually liberates oxygen to kill bacteria in the presence of water. Used for acne. The other effects are keratolytic, comedolytic, mild desquamation to shed comedone caps; reduces production of irritant fatty acids of sebum.

Burning or tingling sensation may be felt. Localized erythema may occur. It should not touch eyes, lips, mucous membranes or denuded skin or hair (may bleach it). Dryness of skin, sealing, sensitization, edema may occur.

Available as 2.5%, 5%, gel or 10% cream.

BENZYL BENZOATE

It is included in WHO and Indian essential medicine list.

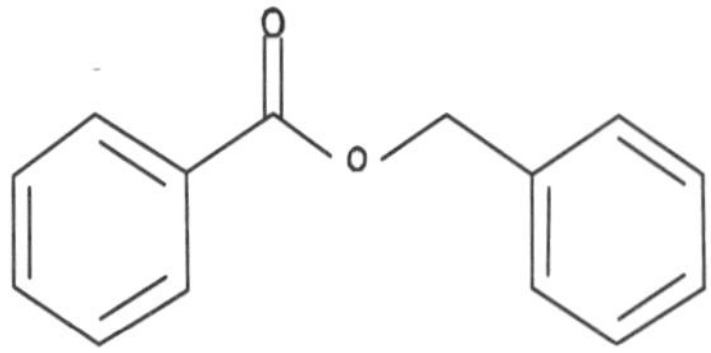

A 25% oily liquid with faint aromatic smell. It is applied for treatment of scabies all over body except face and neck after a soap bath. 2nd application made after 24 hours. It is also effective for pediculosis.

It is minimally absorbed from skin neurological symptoms may appear in children. Contact dermatitis may occur.

BENZYL PENICILLIN (PENICILLIN G)

It is a narrow spectrum antibiotic included in WHO and Indian essential medicine list. It primarily acts on gram positive bacteria.

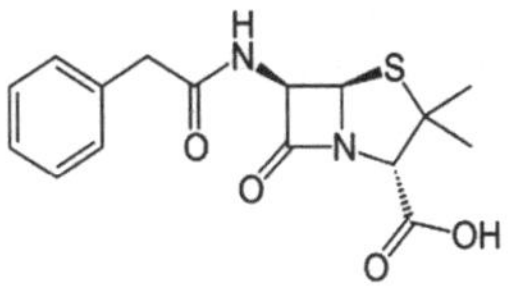

Its spectrum includes *Streptococi, Staph aureus, N.gonorrhoea, N. meningitides, B.anthracis, C. diphtheriae, Clostridia tetani, Listeria, T. pallidum, Actinomycis israelli* are moderately sensitive.

Its primary resistance mechanism is liberation of penicillinase by bacteria.

It is acid labile so destroyed by gastric acid. Reaches most body fluids and excreted by kidney by glomerular filtration and tubular secretion. Tubular secretion in blocked by probenecid, so it prolongs penicillin's action.

Available as crystalline penicillin 0.5-5 M.U. given I.M. or I.V. QDS to BID.

Adverse Effects: Local irritants, Hypersensitivity-Superinfection; Jerisch-Herxheimer reaction.

Uses: Streptococcal, pneumococcal, meningococcal, gonorrhea, syphilis, diphtheria, tetanus, gas gangrene, anthrax, actinomycosis, trench mouth, rat bite fever, listeria monocytogens, Pasteurella multocide.

BETAMETHASONE

It is included in WHO and Indian essential medicine list.

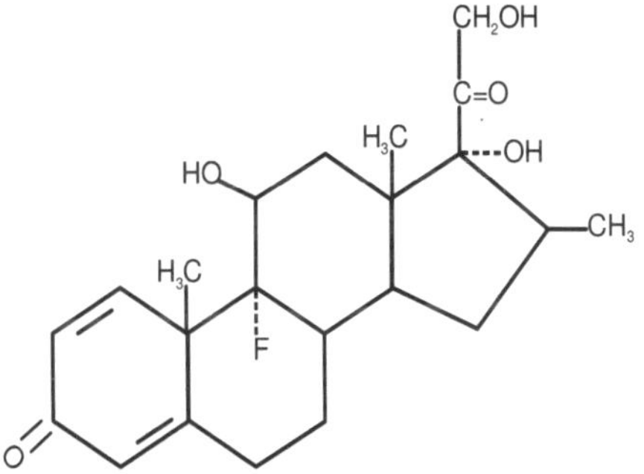

Can be given orally 0.5-5 mg/day; 4-20 mg I.M. or I.V. and applied topically. It is preferred for cerebral oedema and other fluid retentive state.

Available as 0.5 mg and 1 mg tab, 4 mg/ml as (sod. PO_4 salt) for I.M. or I.V. injection 0.5 mg/ml oral drops. 0.025% cream (as benzoate). 0.12% cream (as valerate).

Therapeutic Uses: Systematically: Acute adrenal insufficiency, Rheumatoid arthritis, Rheumatic fever, Collagen diseases (SLE, polyartritis nodosa, Dermatomysitis, nephrotic syndrome), allergic reaction auto immune diseases. In infective diseases with chemotherapeutic cover, topical instillation in eye diseases (allergic conjunctivitis; irits; iridocyclitis), retinitis, uveitis require systemic corticosteroids are required for skin diseases (pemphigus, Stevans-Johnson syndrome, exfoliative dermatitis); cerebral edema; malignancies; septic shock; organ transplantation; thyroid storm; to test adrenal pituitary axis.

ADR: Na and water retention, Cushing's syndrome, hyperglycaemia, susceptible to infection; delayed skin healing; peptic ulcer, osteoporosis, cataract, glaucoma, psychiatric problem, suppression of pituitary adrenal axis, foetal abnormalities, cleft palate.

Adverse effects of topical steroids. Thinning of epidermis; striae; easy bruising; hypopigmentation; delayed wound healing; bacterial and fungal infection.

BETAXOLOL

It is included in Indian essential medicine list.

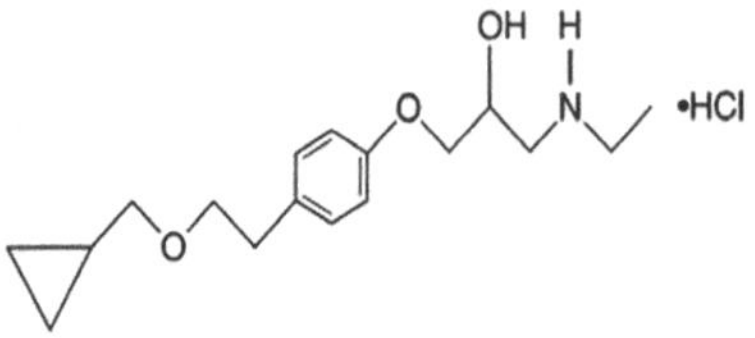

This is selective β_1 receptor blocker used topically to reduce intra-ocular tension in patient of glaucoma. It has less broncho-pulmonary, cardiac, central and metabolic side effects.

Available as 0.5% eye drop.

Stinging and burning sensation of eye may occur.

BIPERIDEN

It is included in WHO essential medicine list.

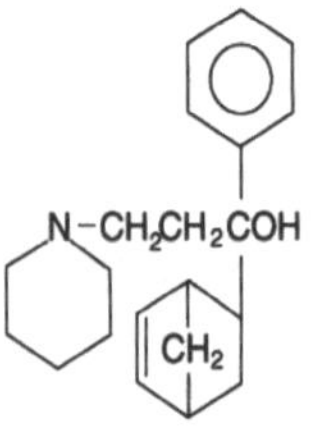

Biperiden is used in the dose of 2-12 mg daily in Parkinsonism. This central antimuscarinic improves tremor and rigidity of Parkinsonism, but its effect on bradykinesia is not that marked.

BISACODYL

It is included in essential medicine list of India.

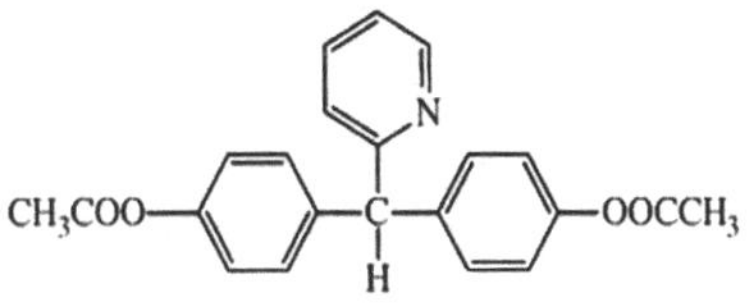

It is a stimulant purgative. It is partly absorbed and re-excreted in bile. It is activated in intestine by deacetylation. It acts on colon to irritate it. Bowel semiformed is evacuated after 6-8 hours.

Available as 5 mg tab, 5 mg tab suppository, acts within 20 minutes.

Mucosa becomes leaky. Stevens-Johnson syndrome, rash, fixed drug eruption may occur.

Used for:

i. Functional constipation.
ii. Atonic constipation.
iii. To bed ridden patient.
iv. To avoid straining of stool.
v. To prepare bowel for surgery, colonoscopy, abdominal X-ray.
vi. With antihelmintic drug.
vii. Food poisoning to drive out the irritants.

BLEACHING POWDER

Ca (OCl) Cl

Bleaching powder is prepared by the action of chlorine on lime producing a mixture of calcium chloride and calcium hypochlorite. It on exposure decomposes to release 30-35% w/w chlorine.

It is used to:

i. Disinfectants of drinking water.
ii. Disinfecting swimming pools, sanitizers or prives.

BLEOMYCIN

Included in WHO and Indian essential medicine list.

Bleomycin is a small peptide. It acts as an anti-cancer drug by binding to DNA which breaks single and double strand DNA following free radical formation and inhibits DNA synthesis.

It is cell cycle specific for G_2 phase. It chelates copper or iron.

Therapeutic Uses:

i. Hodgkin and non-Hodgkin's lymphoma.
ii. Germ cell tumor.

iii. Head and neck cancer.
iv. Squamous cell cancer (skin, cervix; vulva).
v. Sclerosing agent of malignant pleural effusion.

Available as 15 mg inj.

Dose: 30 mg weekly I.M. or I.V. up to 400 mg.

Adverse reaction: Acute: Hypotension, fever, allergic reaction.

Delayed toxicity: Skin toxicity, pulmonary fibrosis, mucocutaneous toxicity, alopecia.

BRETYLIUM TOSYLATE

It is included in essential medicine list of India.

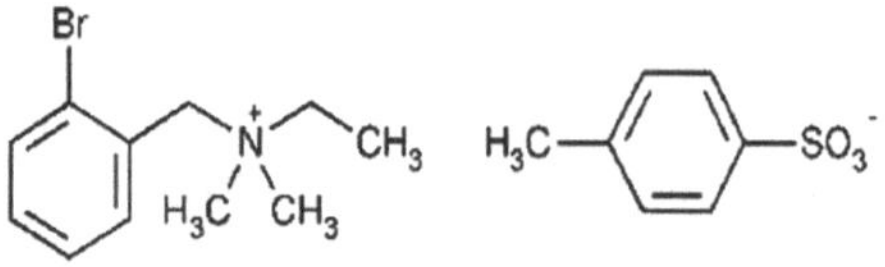

It interferes with neuronal release of catecholamine. Originally introduced as anti-hypertensive but was withdrawn, but reintroduced for parenteral use to facilitate reversal of AF. It increases ventricular but not atrial action potential duration and effective refractory period. Since it may cause initial release of catecholamine causing some inotropic effect in the beginning and may precipitate ventricular arrhythmia. Postural hypotension, nausea, vomiting may occur on I.V. infusion.

Dose: 5 mg/kg over 10 minutes and then constant infusion 0.5-2 mg/kg as maintenance.

BROMOCRIPTINE

Included in Indian essential medicine list.

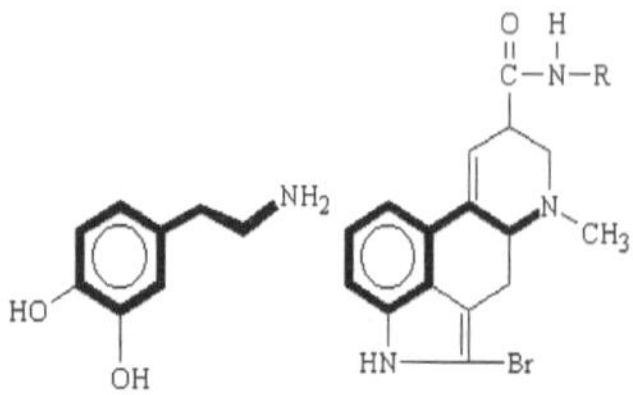

Dopamine Bromocriptine

Chemically it is 2 bromo-alfa ergocriptine is semi-synthetic ergot has dopaminergic action (D_2 action).

It is partial agonist or antagonist to D_1 receptor.

Actions:

i. Decreases prolactin release.
ii. Decrease GH from pituitary tumours.
iii. Antiparkinsonian.
iv. Produces nausea and vomiting.
v. Hypotension.
vi. G.I. motility decreases.

It is partly absorbed from G.I. tract and its metabolites are excreted in bile.

Available as 1.25 mg and 2.5 mg tabs. Start as 1.25 mg BD then increase gradually.

ADR: Nausea, vomiting, nasal blockade, postural hypotension, behavioral change, abnormal movements, livedo reticularis may occur.

Therapeutic Uses:

i. Hyperprolactinemia.
ii. Acromegali.
iii. Parkinsonism.
iv. Hepatic coma.
v. To suppress lactation.
vi. Diabetes mellitus.

BUPIVACAINE

It is included in WHO's and Indian essential medicine list.

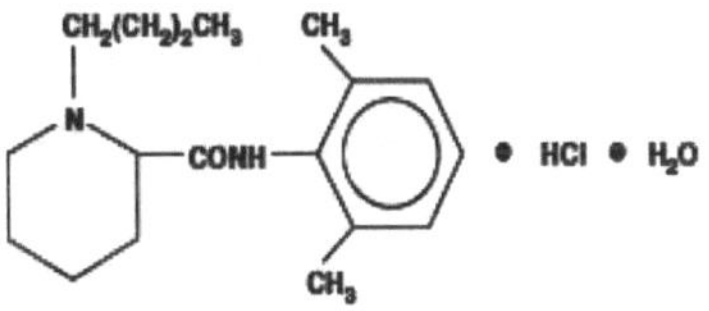

It is amide containing local anaesthetics with high potency and long duration of action. It is used for infiltration, nerve block, epidural, spinal anaesthesia. 0.25%, 0.5% solution injected for obstetrics purpose and for post-operative pain relief.

It is prone to produce prolongation of QT_C interval.

Available as 0.5% and 1% (hyperbaric spinal anaesthesia) S(-) enantiomer is equally potent but less cardio toxic.

BUSULFAN

It is enlisted in essential medicine list of India.

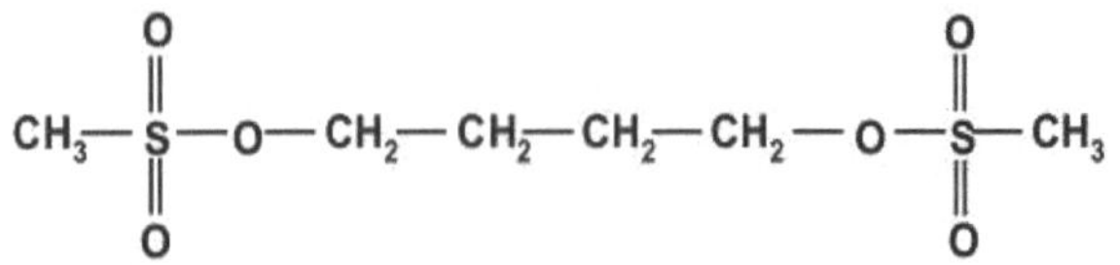

Busulfan is an alkylating agent anti-cancer drug. It is higly effective for myeloid element (granulocyte precursors are sensitive than platelets and RBC).

Pulmonary fibrosis, hyperuricaemia, nausea and vomiting may occur as ADR.

Available as 2 mg tab.

Dose: 2-8 mg/day. Total dose 150-250 mg.

CAFFEINE

It is enlisted in WHO essential medicine list.

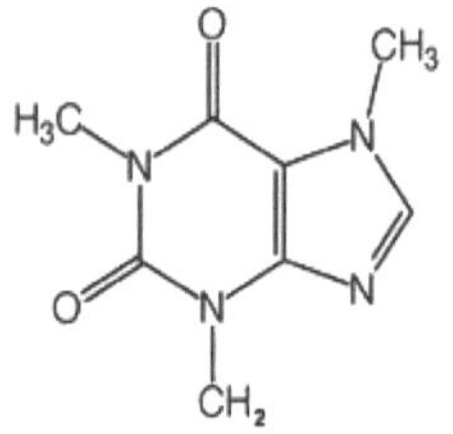

Theophylline, theobromine and caffeine are important methylxanthine, the major source for them are tea, cocoa, coffee respectively. Caffeine is CNS stimulant. It is absorbed from G.I. tract by rapid but irregularly, bound to plasma protein 50%, metabolized in liver by de-methylation and oxidation and then excreted in urine.

ADR: Nausea, vomiting, nervousness, insomnia, agitation, muscle twitching, rigidity, convulsion, rise of temperature may occur tachycardia, extrasystole.

Therapeutic Uses:

i. As analgesic mixture of APC in aspirin + paracetamol +caffeine. Here it allays fatigue and boredom.
ii. Migraine used with ergot. Acting as adjuvant to enhance absorption of ergot and to constrict cranial vessels.
iii. Apnoea in premature infant as alternative to theophylline.

CALAMINE LOTION

It is enlisted in WHO and Indian essential medicine list.

Prepared as following:

Treatment:

Calamine	15 gm (Calamine is zinc oxide with small amout of ferric oxide)
Zinc oxide	5 gm
Bentonite	3 gm
Sodium citrate	0.5 gm
Liquid phenol	0.5 ml
Glycerine	5.0 ml
Rose water	100 ml

Calamine acts as protective and antipruritic. Zinc oxide as astringent. Bentonite acts as protective. Liquid phenol as antiseptic. Glycerine prevents drying of lotion as it is hygroscopic.

CALCIUM GLUCONATE

Enlisted in WHO and Indian essential medicine list.

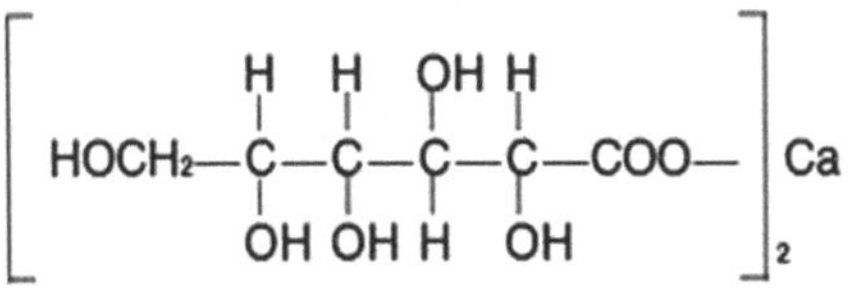

$C_{12}H_{22}CaO_{14}$ **430.38**

Preparation:

Calcium gluconate 9% as calcium is available as 0.5 g and 1 gm tablets and 10% as injection. A sense of warmth is produced on I.V. injection. It does not irritate G.I. tract

Therapeutic Uses:

i. Tetany.
ii. Dietary supplements.
iii. Osteoporosis.
iv. As antacids.
v. Empirically for paraesthesia, weakness and dermatosis.

ADR: Constipation, bloating of abdomen may occur with oral preparation.

CAPREOMYCIN

It is enlisted in WHO's essential medicine list.

Capreomycin is obtained from *Streptomyces capreolus.*

It is peptide protein inhibitor. It is administered deep I.M. As compared to other antibiotics obtained from streptomyces species it is less toxic. It is used for drug resistant tuberculosis 15 mg/kg/day. Resistance may occur due to rrs mutation.

ADR includes : Tinnitus, deafness, vestibular disturbances, nephrotoxicity, local pain, sterile abscess.

It should be dissolved in 2 ml of NaCl injection or sterile water for injection which takes 2-3 minutes for dissolution.

Available as Capreomycin sulfate 0.75, 1gm of capreomycin in 5 ml container.

TRADE NAME: KAPOCIN.

CARBAMAZEPINE

Enlisted in WHO and Indian essential medicine list.

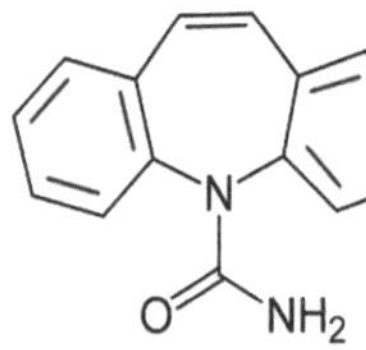

Carbamazepine is tricycle compound. It contains a urede molecule (-N-CO-NH_2) in the heterocyclic ring.

It is orally absorbed, through the rate of absorption varies widely, 70% plasma bound. It induces microsomal enzymes. It is completely metabolized in human to several derivatives one of which is 10, 11 epoxide has anti-convulsant property. Since it induces hepatic microsomal enzymes, it may decrease its level and increases metabolism of other drugs like primidone phenytoin, valproic acid. Some drugs may inhibit its clearance, viz. propoxyphene, trioleandomycin. Protein binding not much interfering in drug interactions.

ADR: Diplopia, Ataxia, Hyponatremia, Water intoxication, G.I. upset, erythematous skin rash, agranulocytosis and blood dyscrasia.

Therapeutic Uses:

i. Complex partial seizure.
ii. Generalized tonic-clonic seizure.
iii. Simple partial seizure.
iv. Trigeminal neuralgia.
v. Cranial diabetes insipidus.
vi. Manic depressive illness and acute mania.

Dose: 200-400 mg TDS; Children 15-30 mg/kg/day.

Available as: 100, 200, 400 mg tabs, 100 mg/5 ml syr.

Also available as sustained or controlled release tablets.

TRADE NAME: TEGRETOL; MAZETOL.

CARBIMAZOLE

Enlisted in Indian essential medicine list.

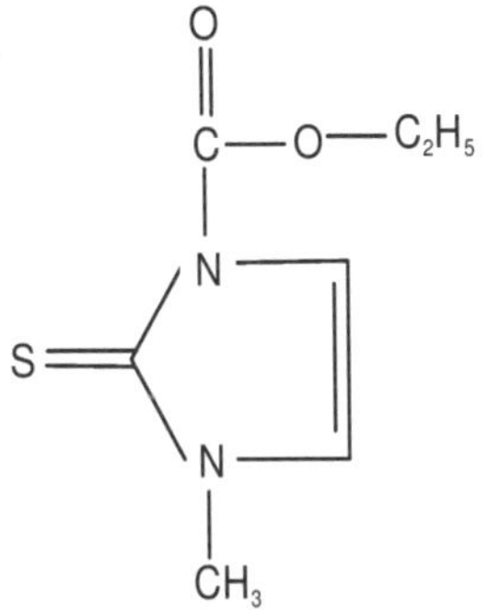

This is an antithyroid drug which inhibits synthesis of thyroid hormones.

These are quickly absorbs orally, with wide distribution (enters milk and placenta), metabolizes in liver and is excreted with urine.

ADR: Hypothyroidism, Goitre, G.I. intolerance, skin rash, Agranulocytosis, graying of hair, loss of taste.

Therapeutic Uses:

i. Thyrotoxicosis, Graves' disease, Toxic nodular goitre.
ii. Pre-operatively in thyrotoxic patient.
iii. Along with I^{131}.

Advantages

i. No surgical risk.
ii. Hypothyroidism is reversible.
iii. Can be given to children.

Disadvantages

Prolonged and unpredictable treatment with chances of drug toxicities.

Available as 5 mg tab.

Dose: 5-15 mg TDS initially then maintenance dose. 2.5-10 mg daily.

TRADE NAME: NEO-MARCAZOLE; THYROZOLE.

CEFAZOLIN

Enlisted in WHO essential medicine list.

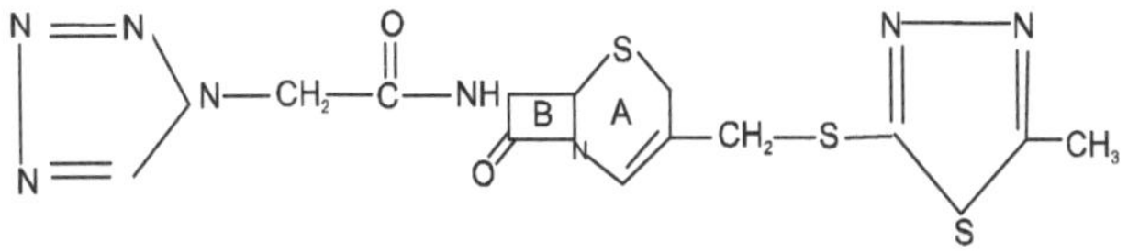

It is 1st generation, per-enterally used cephalosporin.

It is effective against *Strepto* pyogenes, *Strepto* viridans, *Gonococci, Meningococci, Clostridia, H. influenzae, Actinomyces, C. diphtheriae.*

It can be given I.M. or I.V. It is slowly secreted by tubules. It is preferred for surgical prophylaxis.

Dose: 0.25 gm 8 hourly or 1g 6 hourly if infection is severe.

Available as 0.25, 0.5, 1g/vial.

TRADE NAME: ALCIZON; REFLIN.

CEFIXIME

This 3rd generation orally active cephalosporin is included in WHO's essential medicine list.

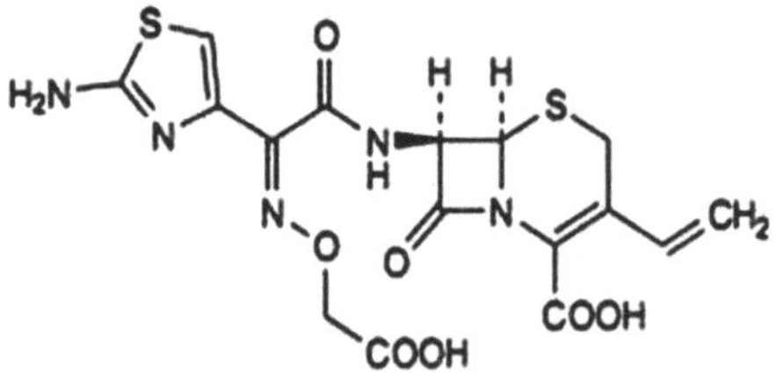

It is highly active against *Enterobactericeae, H. influenzal.* Not active on *Staph aureus, Pneumococcus, Pseudomonas.*

Therapeutic Uses: UTI, RTI, Biliary infection by susceptible organism. Diarrhoea may occur.

Dose: 200-400 mg BD.

Available as 100, 200 mg tab, 100 mg/5 ml syrup.

TRADE NAME: TOPCEF; ORFIX.

CEFOTAXIME

This is 3rd generation perenterally used cephalosporin included in WHO's essential medicine list.

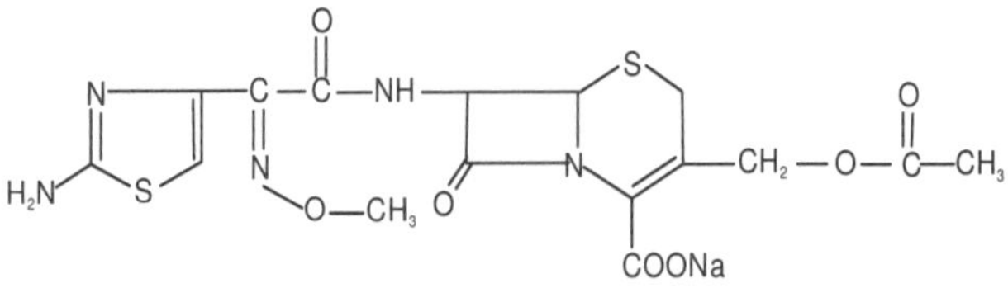

This third generation cephalosporin exerts action on aerobic gram negative and some gram positive bacteria but not active against *Pseudomonas, Anaerobes* and *Staph aureus.*

Used for Meningitis (by gram negative bacilli), Septicemia, hospital acquired infection.

It is given with probenecid as single dose therapy of PPNG urethritis.

It is deacetylated and this metabolite has weaker action. Given 12 hourly because of longer stay of the metabolite in the body.

Dose: 1-2 g I.M. or I.V. 12 hourly.

Children 50-100 mg/kg/day.

Available as 0.25, 0.5 and 1 gm/vial.

TRADE NAME: OMNATAX.

CEFTAZIDIME

This is 3rd generation perenterally used cephalosporin, placed in WHO and Indian essential drug list.

It is effective against *Pseudomonas,* specifically used for febrile neutropenic patient, hematological malignancies, burn, effective against *Enterobacteriacae.*

ADR: Neutropenia, Thrombocytopenia, Rise of BUN and plasma aminotransferase may occur.

Dose: 0.5-2 gm I.M. or I.V. 8 hourly.

Children 30 mg/kg/day.

Typhoid 30 mg/kg.

Available as 0.25, 0.5 and 1 gm vial.

TRADE NAME: FORTUM; ORZID.

CEFUROXIME

This is perenteral 2nd generation cephalosporin, included in Indian essential medicine list.

It is highly effective against PPNG, Ampicillin resistant *H. influenzae.*

It is given I.M. or I.V., attains higher CSF penetration.

Dose: 0.75 g, 1.5 g I.M. or I.V., Children 30-100 mg/kg/day.

Available as 250 mg and 750 mg/vial.

TRADE NAME: CEFOGEN.

Its esters are effective orally. Cefuroxime axetil and its activity depends upon its vivo hydrolysis.

Dose: 250 – 500 mg BD.

Available as 125, 250, 500 mg Cap tab and 125 mg/ 5 ml syrup.

TRADE NAME: CEFTUM; SPIZEF.

CENTCHROMAN

Included in Indian essential medicine list.

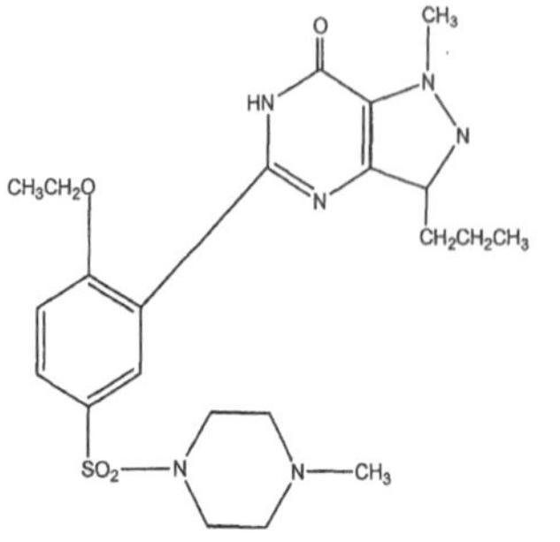

Centchroman is developed in Central Drug Research Laboratory (CDRL), India and introduced in national family welfare programme for O.C.P. This is non-steroidal oestrogen antagonist, probably acts as anti-implantation by producing:

i. Embryo – uterine asynchrony.
ii. Accelerating tubal transport.
iii. Suppression of decidualization.

The conception returns after withdrawal.

ADR: Lengthening and irregular menstrual cycle. No teratogenicity, no abnormal influence on blood sugar, lipid and pituitary ovary endocrine function.

Its plasma t/2 is long about a week.

Dose: 30 mg biweekly × 3 months and then once a week till pregnancy not wanted.

Available as 30 and 60 mg tab.

TRADE NAME: SAHELI; CENTRON.

CEPHALEXIN

This is first generation, orally active cephalosporin included in Indian essential medicine list.

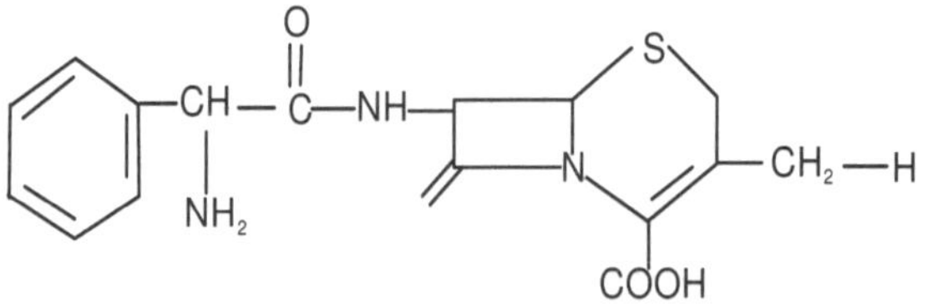

It is effective against gram positive cocci, but less so against penicillinase producing *Staph* and *H. influenzae,* less bound to plasma proteins, bile concentration is high. Excreted unchanged in urine.

Dose: 0.25-1g 6-8 hourly. Children 25-100 mg/kg/day.

Available as 250 mg, 500 mg cap, 125 mg/5 ml dry syrup, 100 mg/ml paediatric drop.

TRADE NAME: SPORIDEX; ALCEPHIN.

CETRIMIDE

It is included in essential medicine list of India.

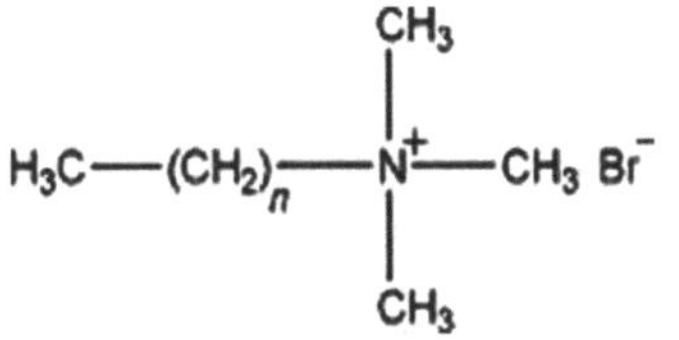

This is creamy white powder, soluble in water. It has bitter and astringent taste. A 0.1 to 1% in water is used as pre-operative disinfectant of skin, applied over denuded skin. A 1:20000 concentration is used for preservative of eye drops. Cream of cetrimide contains 5 g of cetrimide + 50 gms of cetostearyl alcohol + 500 gm of liquid paraffin and made upto 1000 ml with water.

Basically it is surfactants to reduce surface tension of solution also called detergents. Cetrimide is cataonic surfactants with bactericidal activity against gram positive and gram negative organism but relatively ineffective against spores or virus.

Used as antiseptic, disinfectants of surgical instruments, utensils and bath.

Available as CETAVLON.

CHLORAMBUCIL

Included in WHO's essential medicine list.

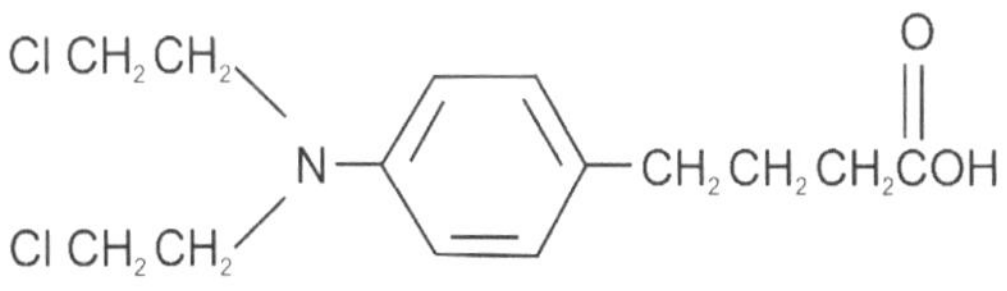

It is used for palliative treatment of CLL, Disseminated Hodgkin's disease (III and IV stages), non-Hodgkin's lymphoma, carcinoma of ovary, breast, mycosis, fungoides, Waldenstrom's microglobulinemia. In combination with methotrexate and dactinomycin used for testicular carcinoma. It is slow acting alkylating agent. It has immune suppressant property.

ADR: Bone marrow depression, Hyperuricaemia.

Available as 2 mg tabs.

Dose: 0.1 – 0.2 mg/kg of body weight daily × 3 to 6 weeks then 2 mg daily. It should be taken 1 hour before breakfast and 2 hours after the evening meal.
TRADE NAME: LEUKERAN.

CHLORAMPHENICOL

It is enlisted in Indian and WHO's essential medicine list.

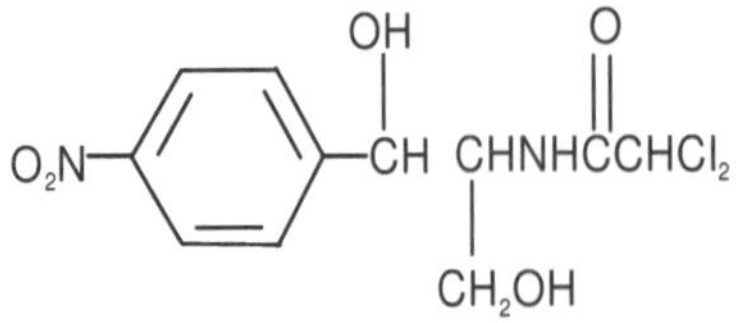

It was initially obtained from *Streptomyces venezuella,* now it is commercially synthetically produced. It is yellowish white crystalline solid with bitter in taste.

It acts on 50s ribosomal subunits and hinders amino acid incorporation. It is bacteriostatic.

Spectrum: *Salmonella, H. influenzae, B. pertussis, Klebsiella, N. meningitidis, Bac. fragilis.*

It is orally active, broad spectrum, 50-60% protein bound, penetrates serous cavities and blood brain barrier. It conjugates with glucuronic acid in liver and excreted unchanged in urine.

ADR: Bone marrow depression, Rash, Atropic glossitis, Nausea, Vomiting, Diarrhea, superinfection, gray baby syndrome in neonates and premature if used in high doses.

Interactions: It inhibits metabolism of tolbutamide, Chlorpropamide, Warfarin, Cyclophosphamide and Phenytoin. Its metabolism is enhanced by phenobarbitone, rifampicin.

Uses: Enteric fever, Pyogenic meningitis, Anaerobic, infection, Intraocular infection.

2nd line treatment of Rickettsia, Whooping cough, U.T.I. Topically used in conjunctivitis or external ear infection.

Available as: 250, 500 mg cap, 0.1% Eye oint, 0.5% Eye drop, 0.5% Ear drops, 1% Applicaps, 125 mg/5 ml oral suspension, 0.25, 0.5, 1 gm/vial injection.

Dose: 250-500 mg 6 hourly, 25-50 mg/kg/day for children. Daily dose should not exceed 2-3 gms and treatment should not exceed 2 weeks.
TRADE NAME: PARAXIN; ENTEROMYCETIN.

CHLORHEXIDINE

Enlisted in WHO and Indian essential medicine list.

It is cationic antiseptic, disrupts bacterial cell wall and denatures microbial proteins. Used as surgical scrub, mouth wash, obstetrics, skin antiseptic, 0.12-2% oral rinse, 0.5-1% tooth paste. It leaves an unpleasant taste and may discolor the teeth. It is biguanide derivative. It is mixible in water.

CHLOROQUINE

Included in WHO and Indian essential medicine list.

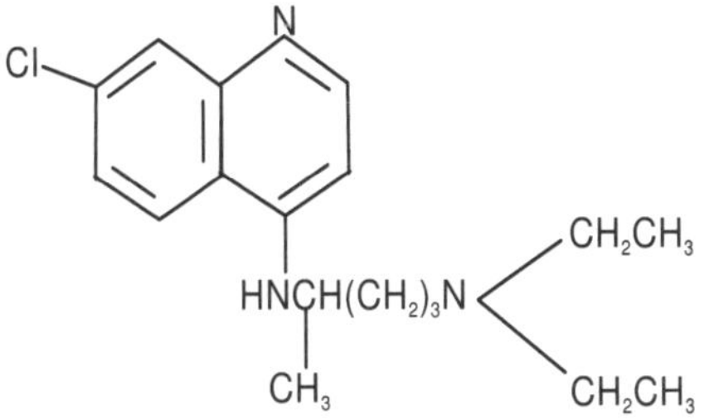

Chloroquine is 4-aminoquinoline. Therapeutically used for:

i. Malaria.
ii. Giardia.
iii. Taeniasis.
iv. Extra intestinal amoebiasis.
v. Chinese liver fluke.
vi. Rheumatoid arthritis.
vii. Discoid lupus and disseminated lupus erythematosus.
viii. Lepra reaction.
ix. Infectious mononucleosis.

It is rapidly and completely absorbed from G.I.T., 55% plasma protein bound, concentrated in liver; spleen, kidney, lung, leukocyte. Degraded in liver microsomal enzymes. Acidification of urine hastens kidney excretion.

ADR: Nausea, Vomiting, Rash, Temporary loss of accommodation with burning of vision diplopia, T wave depression, psychotic episodes, ototoxicity. Used during pregnancy may cause cochleo-vestibular defects, I.V. administration may cause cardiac and respiratory arrest.

Available as chloroquine phosphate 250 mg of salt 1gm followed by 0.5 gm after 6 hours and 0.5 gm daily for 2 days for malaria.

Chloroquine injection NF contains 40 mg of base/ml.

Dose: 200-300 mg of base I.M. in two sites or I.V. slowly.

For children dose should not exceed 5 mg of base/kg.

TRADE NAME: RESOCHIN; LARIAGO.

CHLOROXYLENOL

It is enlisted in WHO essential medicine list.

This antiseptic disinfectant commercially available as 4.8% solution as Dettol, has phenol co-efficient of 70%.

It does not coagulate proteins. It is non-corrosive and non-irritant for intact skin. Poorly water soluble. Used for surgical antisepsis.

Available as cream or soap also. For lubricating obstetric cream (for vaginal examination), as mouth wash. Their activity is decreased if diluted with water and kept for long period.

CHLORPHENIRAMINE

It is included in WHO and Indian essential medicine list.

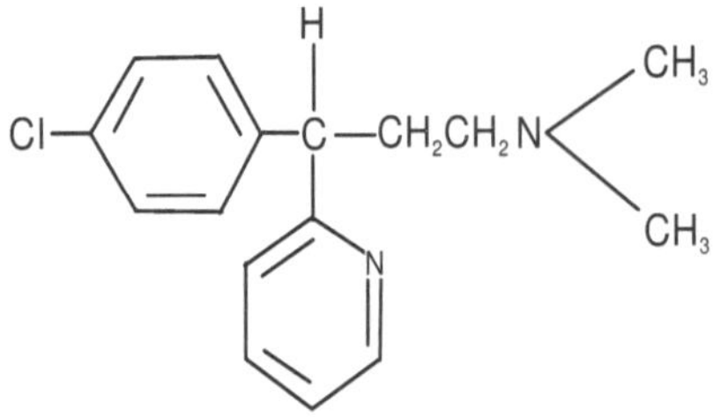

It is orally and perenterally absorbed metabolized in liver and excreted with urine. It is widely distributed in body and enters brain.

ADR: Sedation, diminished concentration, motor incoordination, dry mouth, urinary hesitancy, blurred vision, headache, epigastric distress, contact dermatitis.

Dose: 2-4 mg or 0.1 mg / kg oral or I.M.

Available as PIRITON.

Uses: Anti-allergic: antipruritic, common ingredient of cough remedies.

CHLORPROMAZINE

It is included in both WHO and Indian essential medicine list.

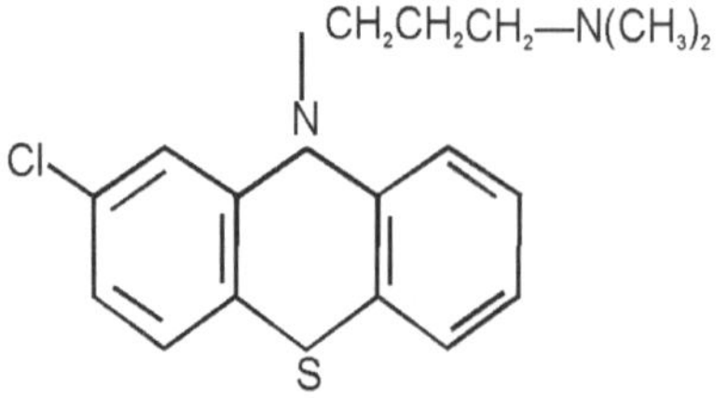

It is the prototype of phenothiazine compounds. It reduces irrational behavior, agitation of psychotics but in normal it produces indifferences in surroundings. It has α-adrenergic properties. Chlorpromazine has local anaesthetic properties too, but it is not used as local anaesthetic because of its irritating properties. It produces hypotension. It increases release. It causes extrapyramidal side effects because it blocks the dopamine receptor in basal ganglion.

Therapeutic Uses:

i. Schizophrenia.
ii. Senile psychosis.
iii. Maniac depressive psychosis.
iv. Antiemetic and antihiccough.
v. Pre-anesthetic medication.
vi. Muscle relaxant in tetanus.

Available as 10, 25, 50, 100 mg tabs. 5 mg/ 5 ml pediatric, 25 mg/5ml adult syrup. 50 mg/2 ml injection. Antipsychotic dose 100-800 mg/day.

TRADE NAME: LARGACTIL / CHLORPROMAZINE.

CHLORTHALIDONE

Included in Indian essential medicine list.

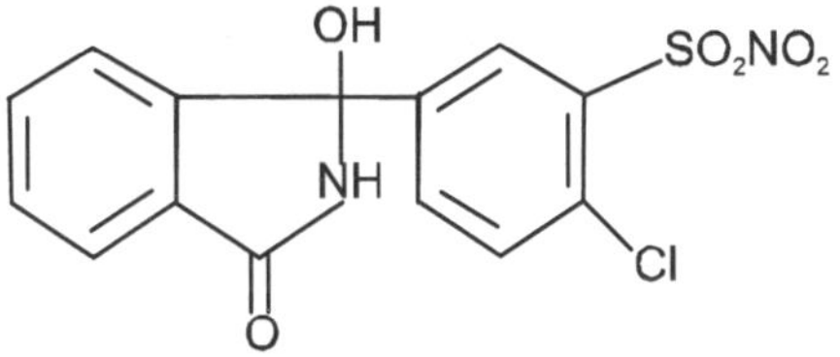

This is thiazide group of diuretics, with medium efficacy inhibits Na^+Cl^- symport. It is orally well absorbed. Action starts within 1 hour. Undergoes hepatic metabolism.

Dose: 50-100 mg at breakfast daily or on alternate day. Maintenance dose should be adjusted. Children 2 mg/kg body weight thrice weekly.

Available as 50 and 100 mg tab.

Therapeutic Uses:

i. Oedema.
ii. Hypertension.
iii. Diabetes insipidus.
iv. Hypercalciuria.

Complications and ADR

i. Hypokalaemia.
ii. Saline depletion.
iii. Nausea, vomiting, diarrhoea.
iv. Hearing loss.

v. Rash, photosensitization.
vi. Hyperuricaemia.
vii. Hyperglycaemia.
viii. Hyperlipidemia.
ix. Mg depletion.
x. Renal failure may aggravate.
xi. Don't use in toxaemia of pregnancy.
xii. Precipitate hepatic coma.

TRADE NAME: HYTHALTON.

CHOLERA VACCINE

Included in WHO's essential medicine list.

Cholera vaccine is phenol or formalin killed suspension of Inaba and Ogawa strains of *V. cholerae* in 5, 10, 30 ml vial. Each ml contains 8×10^9 organisms.

It is given 0.5 ml I.M. or subcutaneous, the second dose is 1 ml after 1-4 weeks. For mass innoculation it is given 1 ml. The protection is 50% and lasts for 6 months so the epidemic is over. Mass innoculation during gathering (melas) does not reduce the incidence because it takes 2-3 weeks to develop immunity after innoculation.

ADR: Fever, aches, pain, local soreness may occur, which may last 1-2 days.

CIPROFLOXACIN

It is enlisted in WHO and Indian essential medicine list.

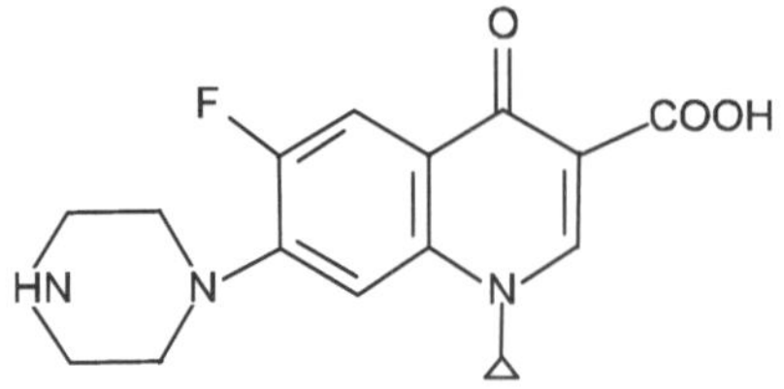

This fluroquinolone inhibits bacterial DNA gyrase to produce its effects.

Resistance develops due to mutation (which reduces affinity of FQ or decreases permeability and increases efflux of FQ across the bacterial membrane.

It is orally absorbed, has high tissue permeability (in lungs, sputum, muscle, bones, prostrates). Excreted with urine by glomerular filtration and tubular secretion.

ADR: Nausea, vomiting, bad taste, dizziness, headache, anxiety, rash, pruritis, photosensitivity, urticaria, tendonitis.

Drug Interactions:

i. It increases theophylline and warfarin level by inhibiting their metabolism.

ii. Its absorption in reduced by antacids and sucralfate.

iii. CNS toxicity is increased by concurrent use with NSAID.

It is contraindicated in pregnancy.

Therapeutic Uses: UTI, gonorrhea, chancroid, gastroenteritis by bacteria, typhoid, R.T.I., bone, soft tissue and gynae infections, tuberculosis, meningitis, gram negative septicaemia, prophylactically in neutropenic and cancer patient, topically in conjunctivitis.

Available as: 250, 500, 750 mg tab 200 mg/100 ml I.V., 3 mg/ml eye drop.

COMMON TRADE NAME: CIFRAN; CIPLOX.

CISPLATIN

Enlisted in WHO and Indian essential medicine list.

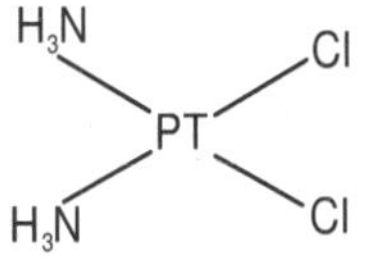

Cisdiamminedichloro platinum kills cells in all stages of cell cycle by binding and formation of inter and intrastrand cross links to inhibit DNA synthesis and functions.

Effective in solid tumours, non small cell and small cell lung cancer, oesophageal cancer, gastric cancer. Head-neck cancer, genitourinary cancers, metastatic ovarian and testicular tumour.

ADR: Vomiting, Renal impairment (Hydrate the patient to reduce it). Deafness, Tinnitus, Neuropathy, Shock like state, Hyperuricaemia.

Dose: 50-100 mg/square meter body surface given I.V. every 3-4 weeks

Available as: 10 mg/10 ml or 50 mg/50 ml vial.

TRADE NAME: CISPLAT; PLATINEX.

CLARITHROMYCIN

Enlisted in Indian essential medicine list.

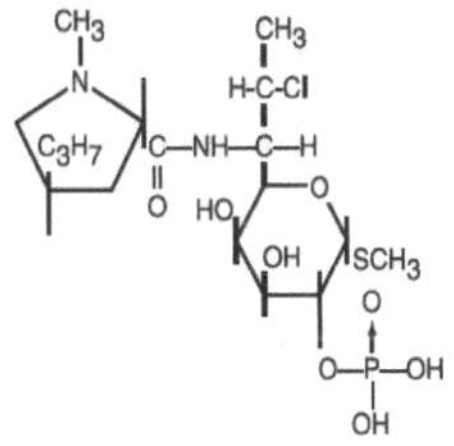

Clarithromycin is macrolide antibiotic which is derived from erythromycin by addition of methyl group which improves its acid stability and oral absorption in comparison to erythromycin. It is also effective against Mycobact avium complex (MAC) and other atypical mycobacteria, *Mycobact leprae, H. pylori, Moraxella, Legionella, Mycoplasma pneumonae.* The bacteria which has developed resistance to erythromycin is resistance to this antibiotic also. It is indicated in upper and lower RTI, sinusitis, otitis media, whooping cough, skin infections, H. pylori infection, MAC, leprosy.

It is rapidly absorbed, 50% bioavailable. Its absorption is delayed by food, produces active metabolite and excreted unchanged with urine.

Dose: 250 to 500 mg BD for 7-14 days.

Available as 250, 500 mg tabs; 125 mg/5 ml and 250 mg/5 ml syrup.

ADR: Hearing loss, pseudomembranous colitis, hepatic dysfunction, rhabdomyolysis are important side effects, other than those of erythromycin, safety in pregnancy and lactation is not known.

TRADE NAME: CLARIBID/CLARIMAC.

CLINDAMYCIN

It is enlisted in WHO essential medicine list.

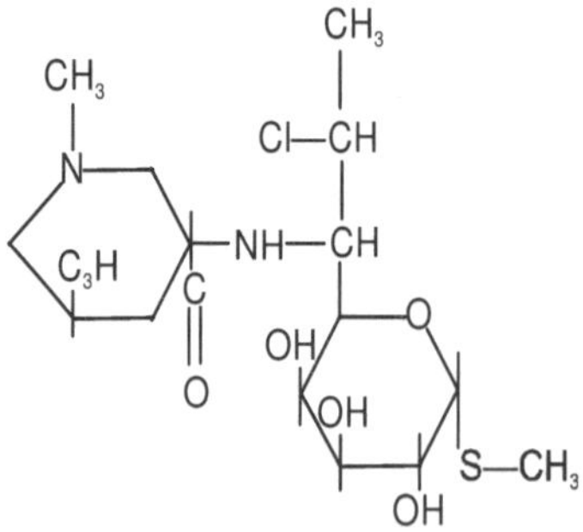

Which is chlorine substituted derivative of lincomycin. It inhibitis protein synthesis by binding 50 S ribosomes.

Spectrum: *Strepto, Staph, Pneumo, C.diphtheriae, Nocardia, Actinomyces, Bact. fragilis.*

It is orally absorbed, 90% protein bound, penetrates all tissues, but penetration in brain is poor. It is metabolized in liver and both the active drug and metabolites are excreted in bile and urine.

Therapeutic Uses: Anaerobic infection caused by bacteroides specially Bact. fragilis causing abdominal pelvic and lung abscess,

Cl. perfringens infection, prophylaxis in bacterial endocarditis patient, Toxoplasmosis patient with pyrimethamine, in pneumocystis jiroveci pneumonia with primaquin.

ADR: Diarrhoea, nausea, skin rash, liver function impairment, enterocolitis, neutropenia.

Dose: 150–300 mg QID orally or 200-600 mg I.V. 8 hourly.

Available as 150, 300 mg cap, 300 mg/2 ml or 600 mg/4 ml vial, 1% Topical solution or gel.

TRADE NAME: CLINCIN; DALCAP.

CLOFAZAMINE

Included in WHO and Indian essential medicine list.

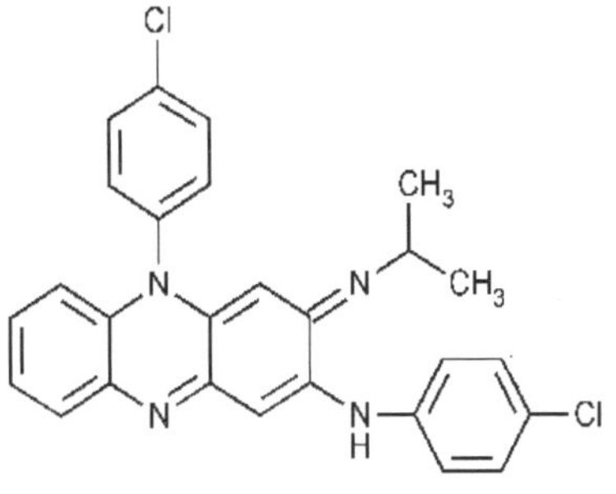

Basically clofazamine is a dye with leprostatic and anti-inflammatory properties. Dapsone resistant leprosy responds to it.

It is orally active, accumulates in many tissues, fat. Its t/2 is 70 days. Used for lepra reaction and in multi-drug therapy of leprosy.

ADR: Reddish black pigmentation of skin, discolouration of skins, acneform eruption, conjunctival pigmentation, loose motion, weight loss, anorexia. It is advisable to avoid it in liver, kidney diseases and in pregnancy.

CLOMIPHENE

Included in WHO and Indian national essential medicine list.

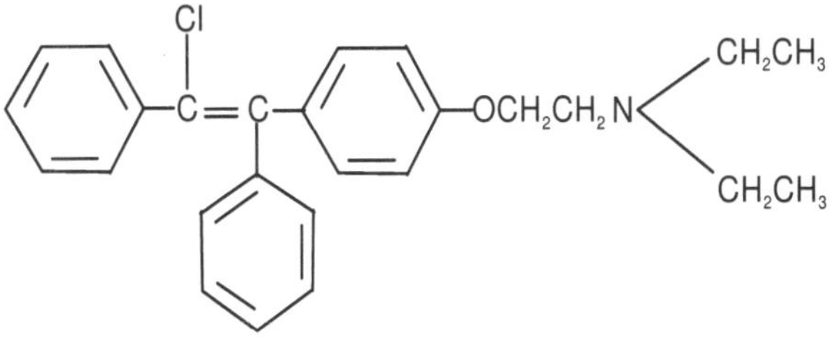

Clomiphene citrate is non-steroidal agent chemically related to chlorotrianisene and triparanol. It acts to ERα and ERβ acts as pure estrogen antagonist in all human tissues. It induces Gn secretion as a consequence of oestrogenic negative feedback inhibition.

Therapeutic Uses:

i. Sterility due to ovulatory failure.
ii. To aid in vitro fertilization.
iii. Oligospermia.

ADR: Multiple pregnancies, polycystic ovaries, hot flushes, vertigo, gastric upset, allergic rhinitis, risk of ovarian tumor.

Available as 25, 50, 100 mg tab.

Dose: 50 mg OD × 5 days from 5th day of cycle.

TRADE NAME: CLOMID; CLOME.

CLOMIPRAMINE

It is included is WHO and Indian essential medicine list.

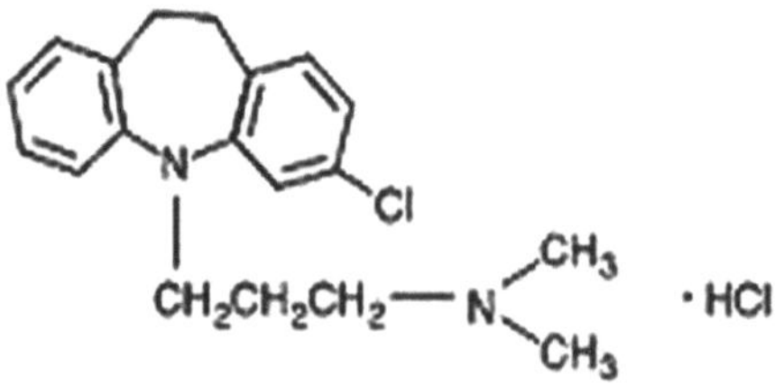

This tricycle anti-depressant inhibits noradrenaline and 5HT reuptake and increases their concentration at synaptic cleft. It is given in the dose of 75-300 mg. It causes sedation, dryness of mouth, fall in BP, cardiac arrhythmia. It may precipitate seizure.

Available as 10, 25, 50 mg tab and 75 mg SR tab.

TRADE NAME: CLOFRANIL; CLONIL.

CLOTRIMAZOLE

It is included in WHO's essential medicine list.

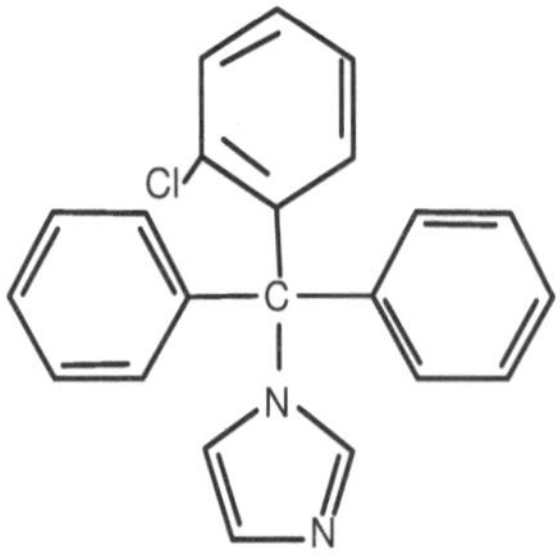

This broad spectrum antifungal drug used topically. Its spectrum includes *Allescheria boydii, Sporotrichum, Histoplasma,*

Blastomyces, Cryptococcus, C. immitis, Aspergillus Candida Dermatophytes *(Epidermophyton, Microsporum, Trichophyton), or Malassezia* furfur.

ADR: It is well tolerated. Topical use may produce erythema, stinging, blistering, peeling, edema pruritis. Oral administration may produce abdominal pain, nausea, vomiting, diarrhoea. It is not intended for ophthalmic use.

Available in India as: 1% lotion, cream, powder, 100 mg vaginal tab.

TRADE NAME: SURFAZ; CLODERM.

CLOXACILLIAN

It is included in both WHO and Indian essential medicine list.

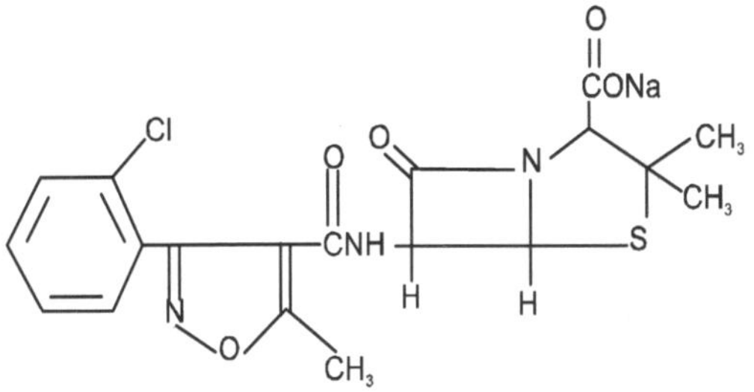

This semi-synthetic penicillin salt is highly penicillinase and acid resistant.

It is orally absorbed, better if taken in empty stomach, 90% plasma protein bound, eliminated by kidney and partly by liver.

Used for mixed infection caused by penicillin G resistant Staph, β-haemolytic strepto and pneumo. Generally well tolerated.

ADR: Rash, diarrhoea, nausea, vomiting, eosinophilia, leukopenia, rise in SGOT: super-infection.

Dose: 0.25-0.5 gm QDS orally or 0.25 to 1 gm I.M. or I.V.

Available as 0.25 gm, 0.5 gm caps 125 mg/3 ml syrup, 0.25 gm and 0.5 gm/vial injection.

TRADE NAME: KLOX.

COAL TAR

Enlisted in WHO and Indian essential medicine list.

Coal tar containing several phenolic compounds, exerts phototoxic effect on skin when exposed to ultraviolet rays and decreases epidermal turnover.

Therapeutic Uses: Applied over psoriatic plaque.

ADR: Bad smell, inacceptable, skin irritation, allergy, photosensitization and carcinogenicity.

Available is combination of salicylic acid 3%, sulfur precipitate 3% and coal tar 6%.

TRADE NAME: EXETAR.

CODEINE

Included both in WHO and Indian essential medicine list.

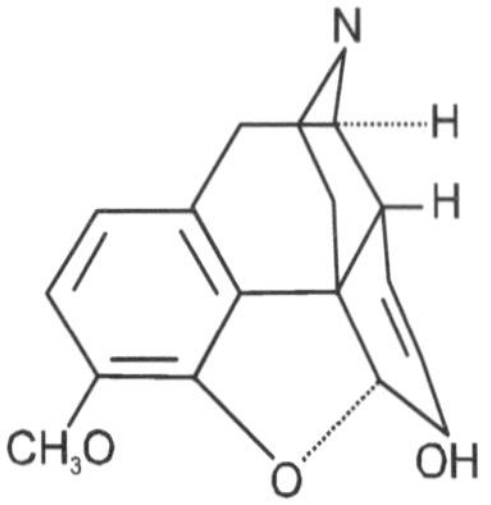

Codeine is considered to be most useful narcotic anti-tussive agent. It belongs to phenanthrene group obtained from milky exudate of poppy seed capsule of the plant *Papaver somniferum*. It is much less potent analgesic than morphine. It is partial agonist of mu(μ) opiod receptor. It is orally active.

ADR: Constipation; Abuse potential.

Therapeutic Uses: Antitussive; to control diarrhoea.

Dose: 10-30 mg for adults; 2.5-5 mg for children of 2–6 years.

Available as 15 mg tab; 15 mg/5 ml linctus.

TRADE NAME: CODEINE 15 mg tab.

COLCHICINE

Enlisted in WHO and Indian essential medicine list.

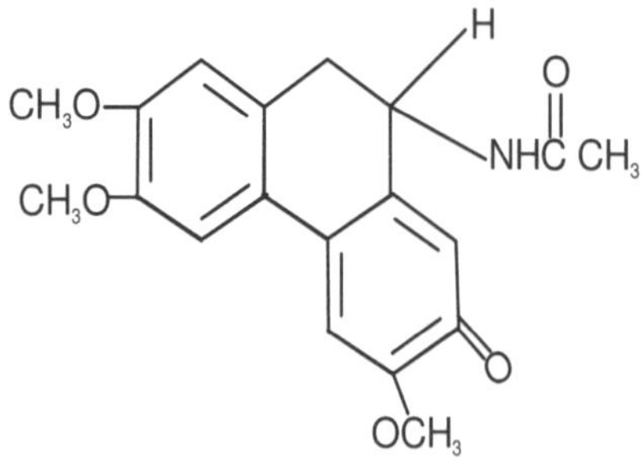

Colchicine is drug of choice of acute gout. Oral administration should start as soon as first sign appears and to continue till symptoms subsides or G.I. distress appears.

It is orally absorbed, metabolized in liver, excreted with bile, undergoes enterohepatic circulation and ultimately excreted with urine and faeces.

ADR: Nausea, vomiting, watery diarrhoea, abdominal cramps, kidney damage, CNS depression, muscular paralysis and respiratory failure, agranulocytosis, should be used with caution in elderly, debilitated with kidney, cardiovascular and G.I. tract diseases.

Bone marrow depression occurs with I.V. administration.

Dose: For acute gout 0.5 or 0.6 mg, administered hourly till symptoms disappears or G.I. upset starts.

Intravenous: 1 to 2 mg initially, then 0.5 mg every 3 to 6 hours, total dose should not exceed 4 mg.

Available as 0.5 mg tab. Or 0.5 mg/ml in 2 ml container.
TRADE NAME: As generic in USA. COLCHINDON tabs.

CONCENTRATED VITAMIN A

Enlisted both in WHO and Indian essential medicine list.

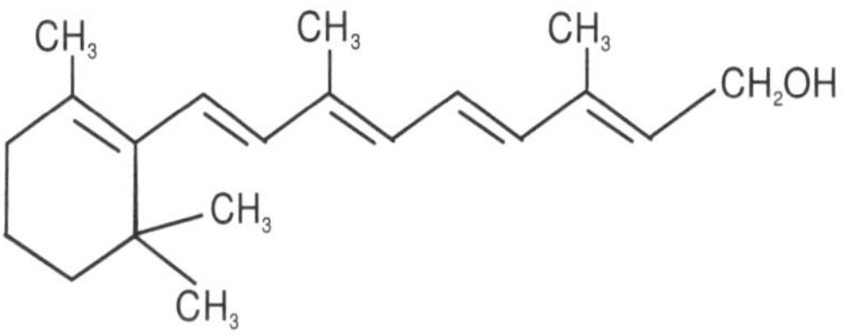

Vitamin A is an unsaturated fat soluble alcohol, essential for growth, bone development in children, for vision in dim light, for integrity of skin and mucous membrane.

Deficiency Symptoms: Phrynoderma, hyperkeratinization, atrophy of sweat glands, xerosis, Bitot's spot, keratomalacia, night blindness, corneal opacitis, diarrhea, urinary stone formation, keratinization of broncho-pulmonary epithelium with infection, sterility, abortion, foetal malformation, growth retardation, impairment of special senses.

Therapeutic Uses: Prophylaxis to vitamin A deficiency in pregnancy lactation, infancy hepatobiliary disease. Treating Vit A deficiency, 50000-100000 I.U., I.M. or orally. In diseases of skin (viz. psoriasis, icthiosis).

Hypervitaminosis of vit A produces (100000 I.U./day × month), nausea, vomiting, itching, exfoliation, loss of appetite, irritability, raised intracranial pressure, bleeding etc. Daily intake should not increase 20000 I.U. It is treated by stopping further intake and with vitamin E.

Preparations:

Injection 50000 I.U./ml in 5 ml container.
Capsules 25000 and 50000 I.U. capsules.
Drops 50000 I.U./ml in 30 ml container.

CO-TRIMOXAZOLE

(Combination of Sulfamethoxazole and Trimethoprim)

Included in the essential medicine list of both WHO and India.

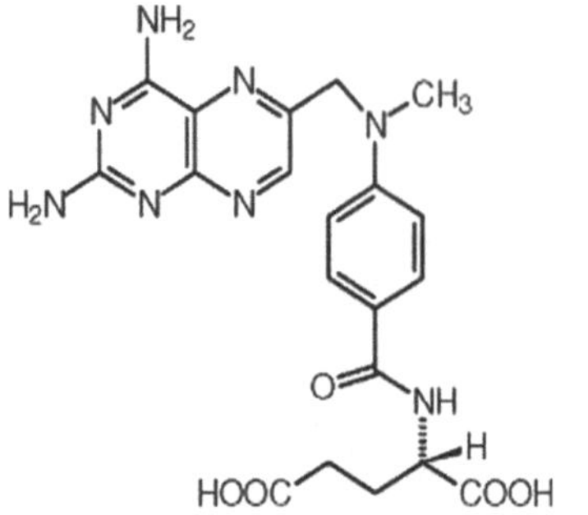

It is a fixed drug combination sulfamethoxazole and trimethoprim in the ratio of 5:1 to block the production of tetrahydrofolic acid from PABA in the bacteria where these two produces sequential block.

Spectrum of the Combination: Salmonella, Serratia klebseilla, Enterobacter, Yersenia, Puterocolitica, Pneumocystis jiroveci, Staph aureus, Strep pyogenes shigella, E. coli, H. influenzae, Gono and meningcoccus

Resistance: Occurs by mutation and plasmid mediated.

ADR: Nausea, vomiting, stomatitis, megaloblastic anemia, blood dyscrasia, neonatal haemolysis.

Uses: UTI, RTI, Typhoid, Bacterial diarrhea and dysentry (by Campylobacter, E coli, shigella), Pneumocystis jiroveci, chancroid.

Available as: Trimethoprim 80 mg and Sulfamethoxazole 400 mg as tab, syrup and injection (per 5 ml).

I.V. preparation is WK TRIM, I.M. preparation is ORIPRIM I.M. TRADE NAME: SEPTRAN.

CYCLOPHOSPHAMIDE

This anti-cancer drug is enlisted in WHO and Indian essential medicine list.

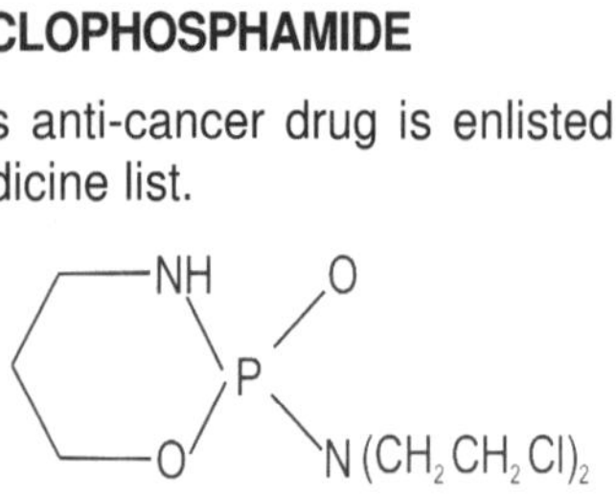

It is an alkylating agent, inactive as such, transformed to active metabolites (Aldophosphamide, phosphoramide mustard) in liver. It has got wide range of anti-cancer activity and prominent immunosuppressant property. Its thrombocytopenic effect is less but alopecia and hemorrhagic cystitis are common (produced by one metabolite acrolein). Its metabolism is retarded by chloramphenicol. Nausea and vomiting are acute toxicities.

Doses: 3.5-5 mg/kg orally, 1 g/m^2 or 10 – 15 mg/kg I.V. per 7 - 10 days.

Available as 50 mg tab, 200, 500, 1000 mg inj.

TRADE NAME: ENDOXAN.

CYCLOSERINE

It is enlisted is WHO's essential medicine list.

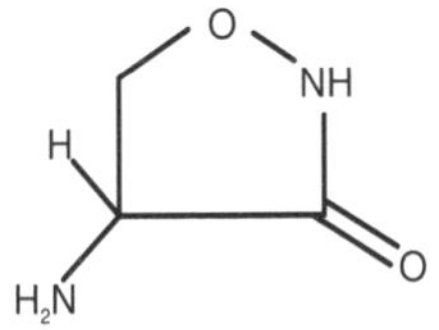

This antibiotic is produced by *Streptomyces orchidaceous.* It is water soluble, unstable in acid pH. It inhibits incorporation of D-alanine in peptidoglycan of bacteria by inhibiting alanine racemase.

It is widely distributed and excreted with urine.

It is effective against mycobacteria and gram negative bacteria.

ADR: Dose related CNS toxicities like headache, tremor, psychosis and convulsion, which can be prevented with pyridoxine (100 mg/day). These CNS effects are low if dose used is below 0.75 gm/day.

Dose: 250 mg BD may be increased upto 500 mg BD, if patient can tolerate it.

Available as: 250 mg capsule.

TRADE NAME: CYCLORINE.

CYCLOSPORINE

Enlisted both in WHO and Indian essential medicine list.

This drug is immunosuppressive through regulation of gene transcription. It inhibits interleukin 1 and interleukin 2 receptor production. It affects T cell dependent B. function.

It is incompletely absorbed. Its absorption is increased if taken with grape juice. It is metabolized by CYP 3A so produces large number of drug interaction.

Therapeutic Uses: Rheumatoid arthritis, SLE, Polymyositis, Dermatomyositis, Wegener's granulomatosis, uveitis, bronchial asthma, inflammatory bowel disease, juvenile chronic arthritis, human organ transplantation to treat graft vs host reaction.

ADR: Nephrotoxicity, Hypertension, Hyperglycaemia, liver dysfunction, hyperkalemia, seizure, altered mental status, Hirsutism, Lymphoma, Kaposi's sarcoma and skin cancer are reported.

Dose: 3-5 mg/kg/day I.V. in divided doses or 10-15 mg/kg /day with grape juice for 1-2 weeks gradually reduced to 2-6 mg/kg.

Available as 25, 50, 100 mg soft gelatin caps, 100 mg/ml in 1 ml, 5 ml, 50 ml vial.

TRADE NAME: IMUSPORIN Caps; SANDIMMUN Injection.

CYTOSINE ARABINOSIDE/CYTARABINE

Included both in WHO and Indian essential medicine list.

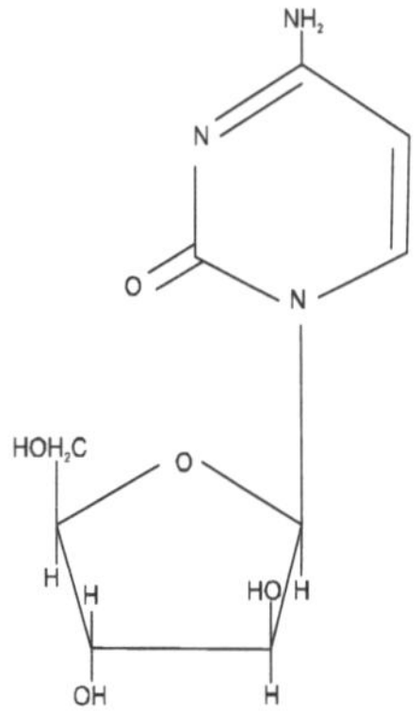

It is pyrimidine antagonist, phosphorylated into the body to corresponding nucleotide to inhibit DNA synthesis and interferes DNA repair. It acts on S phage of cell cycle.

Therapeutic Uses: Remission of acute leukemia, Hodgkin's and non-Hodgkin's lymphoma.

Dose: 1.5-3 mg I.V. BD × 5-10 days.

Available as 100, 500, 1000 mg inj.

TRADE NAME: CYTABIN.

D.P.T. VACCINE

Enlisted both in WHO and Indian essential medicine list.

This is a combination of diphtheria and tetanus toxoid with pertussis vaccine. It is the recommended preparation for primary immunization and recall or booster immunizations in children below 6 years of age. It is available in fluid form and also in precipitated adsorbed form. The adsorbed form is slowly absorbed and is better immunogenic. This combined preparation in not administered after 6 years of age because of severe local and generalized reactions. Tetanus and diphtheria adult type is used after that age.

ADR: Fever, Tenderness, Erythema, convulsion, screaming hypsarrhythmia, Pseudotumor, cerebri or acute disseminated encephalomyelitis.

Any CNS reaction is contraindication of pertussis vaccination.

Dose: 0.5 ml I.M., 2-3 injection in 4-6 weeks apart and booster after year and then at school entry.

Available as TRIPVAC diphtheria toxoid 25 LF, tetanus toxoid 5 LF, B. pertussis 20000 million 0.5 ml amp.

DACARBAZINE

Included in WHO's essential medicine list.

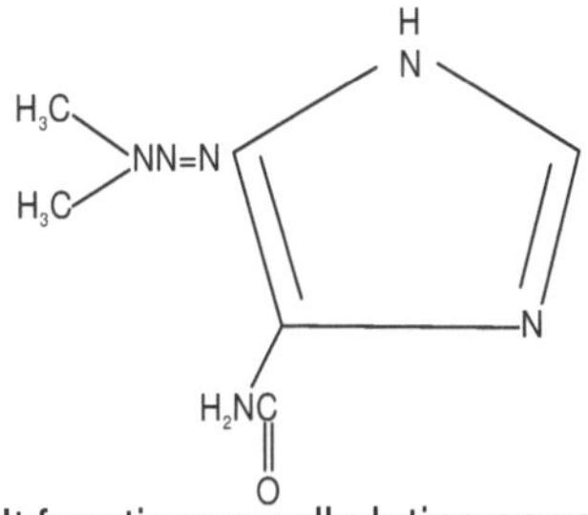

It functions as alkylating agent after metabolic activation in the liver, particularly useful to treat malignant melanoma. Its primary inhibitory action is on RNA protein synthesis. It is also useful for Hodgkin's disease.

Dose: 3.5 mg/kg/day I.V. for 10 days and to be repeated after 4 weeks.

Available as 100, 200, 500 mg inj.

TRADE NAME: DACARIN; DACARZINE.

DANAZOL

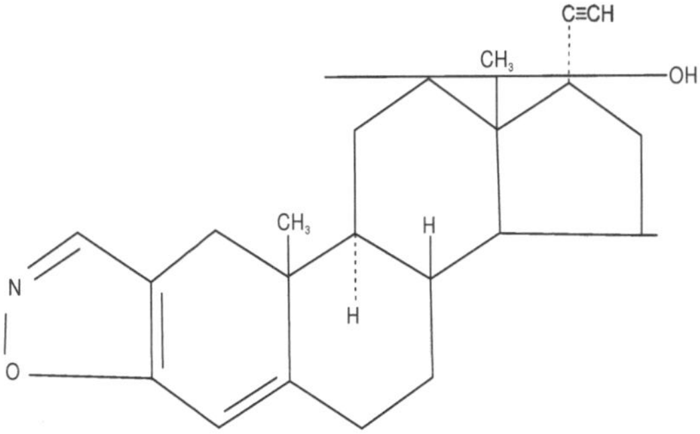

This is synthetic derivative of 17 α-ethynyl testosterone (ethisterone) with weak androgenic anabolic and progestational activities. It is called impeded androgen, because it binds to androgen receptor and induces some of the androgen specific mRNA production. It suppresses Gn secretion from pituitary and inhibits testicular and ovarian function indirectly and directly. Endometrium atrophies.

ADR: Weight gain, Flushing sweating, Vaginitis, acne, hirsutism, oily skin, decreased in breast size. Should not be given in pregnancy, Elevation of liver enzymes, Loss of libido in men.

Therapeutic Uses:

i. Endometriosis.
ii. Menorrhagia.
iii. Fibrocystic breast diseases.
iv. Infertility.
v. Hereditary angioneurotic oedema.

Dose: 200–600 mg/day.

Available as 50,100,200 mg cap.

TRADE NAME: DANAZOL; GONABLOK.

DAPSONE

Included both in WHO and Indian essential medicine list.

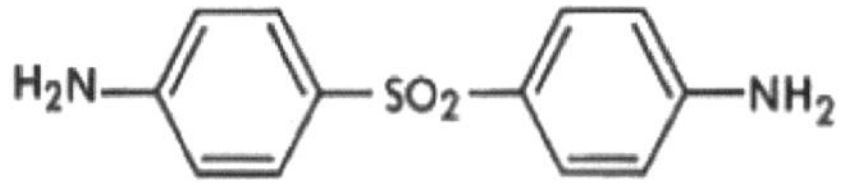

This sulfone is the drug of choice of all forms of leprosy. It is chemically related to sulfonamide and inhibits PABA's incorporation into folic acid. It is leprostatic. The dapsone resistant has started and necessitated the use of MDT i.e. multi drug therapy. It may be primary resistant or secondary resistant.

It is orally completely absorbed, widely distributed except in CSF, 70% protein bound, concentrated more on lepromatous skin. It is acetylated and conjugated with glucuronide and sulfate in liver. These metabolites are excreted with bile and reabsorbed from intestine and ultimately excreted with urine. It is cumulative.

ADR: Haemolytic anaemia, Nausea, Anorexia, Methaeglobin, anemia, Headache, Paraesthesia, Drug fever, Allergic rashes, Hypermelanosis, Exfoliative dermatitis, Phototoxicity.

Therapeutic Uses:

i. Leprosy.
ii. Anti malarial.
iii. Dermatoses (Pyoderma gangrenosum).

Dose: 200 to 300 mg/day.

Available as: 25, 50, 100 mg tab.

TRADE NAME: DAPSONE.

DAUNORUBICIN

Enlisted in WHO's essential medicine list.

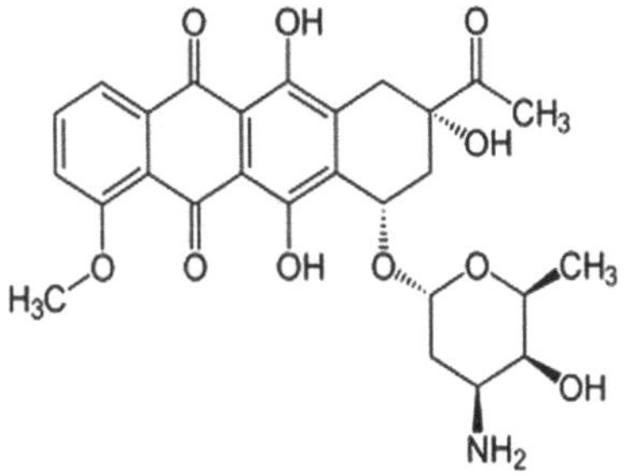

It is an anthracycline antibiotic obtained from *Streptomyces peucetius var caesius.* It inhibits topoisomerase II and intercalates DNA and inhibits its synthesis. It alters fluidity and ion transport and generates semiquinone type free radicals.

It is given I.V., metabolized in liver with reduction and hydrolysis of ring substitution. Hydroxylated metabolite is active and aglycone is inactive.

ADR: Cardiotoxicity, Arrhythmia, Hypotension, CCF, Bone marrow depression, Alopecia, stomatitis, vomiting, local tissue damage if extravasation.

Therapeutic Uses: Cancer breast, endometrium, ovary, testicles, bladder, liver, lung, soft tissue sarcoma, Ewing sarcoma, neuroblastoma, osteosarcoma.

Available as 20 mg/vial inj.

Dose: 30-60 mg/sq meter I.V. × 3 days.

TRADE NAME: DAUNOCIN; DAUNOMYCIN.

DEFEROXAMINE

Enlisted in WHO and Indian essential medicine list.

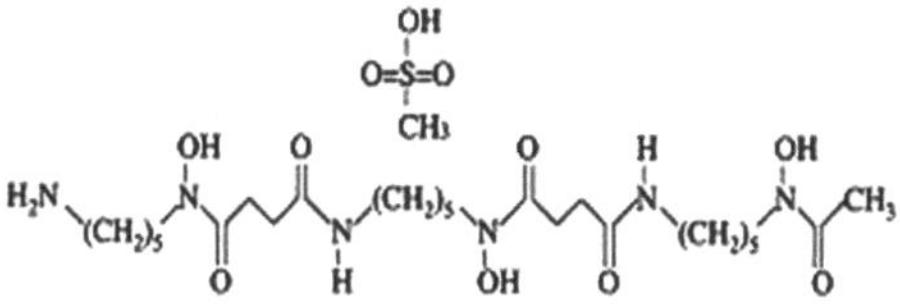

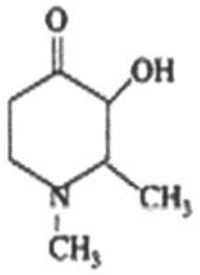

It is obtained from micro organism, *Streptomyces pilosus*. It is highly specific iron chelating agent. It readily complexes with ferric ion and has some affinity for ferrous ion. 1gm of chelator can chelate upto 85 mg of elemental iron. It is straight chain molecule winds round ferric iron and forms a stable non-toxic complex which is excreted with urine. It also removes loosely bound iron and that from haemosiderin and ferratin, but it cannot remove iron from haemoglobin or cytochrome. It has low affinity for calcium when given perenterally. It is partly metabolized and little is absorbed from orally administered.

Therapeutic Uses:

i. Iron poisoning.
ii. Transfusion.
iii. Siderosis.

Dose: 0.5 – 1 g / day I.M. or I.V. with blood transfusion, 2 g/unit of blood transfusion.

ADR: Hypotenision, flushing, itching, urticaria, rash (due to histamine release), abdominal pain, loose motion, muscle cramps, fever, dysuria changes in lens and retina.

Available as 0.5 g/vial.

TRADE NAME: DESFERAL.

DEXAMETHASONE

Enlisted in WHO and Indian essential medicine list.

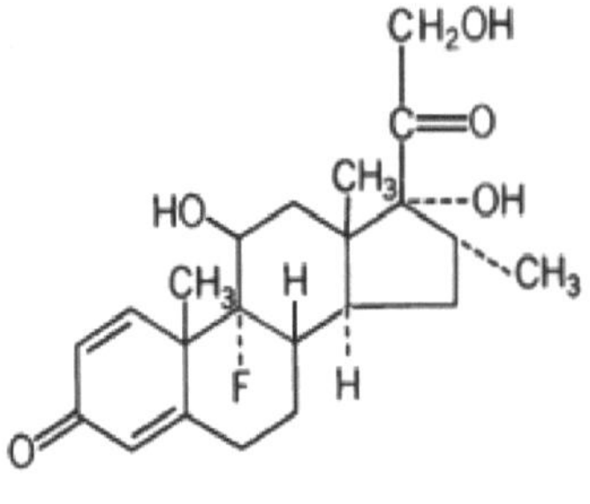

It is fluorinated prednisolone derivative used for inflammatory, allergic and other glucocorticoid responsive diseases. It is very potent, highly selective, long acting glucocorticoids with marked pituitary adrenal suppression. Fluid retention and hypertension is not that problem.

Dose: 0.5 -5 mg/day oral; for allergic condition. 4-20 mg/day I.M. or I.V. infusion for shock and cerebral oedema.

Available as 0.5 mg tab; 4 mg/ml injection. 0.5 mg/ml oral drops. Topical, ophthalmic uses are also there.

TRADE NAME: DECADRON; DEXONA; DECDAN.

DEXTRAN 40 AND 70

Enlisted in Indian essential medicine list.

Dextran 70 in enlisted both in WHO and Indian essential medicine list.

Dextran is a polysaccharide obtained from sugar beat available in two forms 70 (MW 70000) and 40 (MW 40000).

It has all properties of a plasma expander, viz.

i. Exert oncotic pressure comparable to plasma.
ii. Remain in plasma for long time.
iii. Pharmacologically inert and pyrogenic.
iv. Easily sterilizable.
v. Can be stored for 10 years and cheap.

ADR: May interfere grouping and may be antigenic. Dextran 40 acts more rapidly, decreases blood viscosity.

Dose: 20 mg/kg in 24 hours.

Therapeutic Uses: Burns, shock (hypovolumic and endotoxin) trauma, tissue damage, temporary measure of whole blood loss till blood transfusion in arranged.

Contraindications: Anemia, CCF, Pulmonary oedema, Renal insufficiency.

DEXTROMETHORPHAN

Enlisted in Indian essential medicine list.

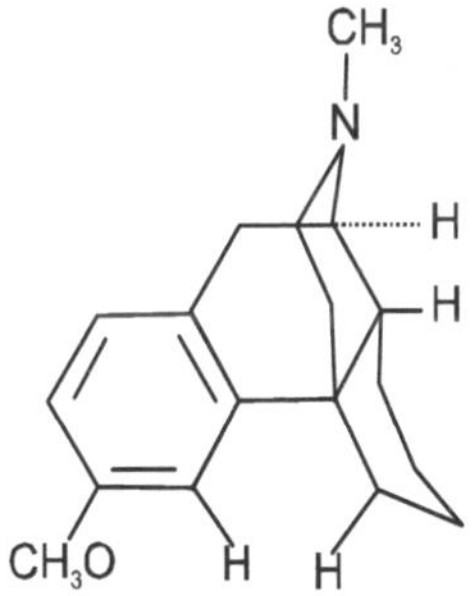

It is methyl either of dextroisomer of the narcotic analgesic levorphanol used as anti-tussive (raises threshold for cough). Constipating effect is less. Suppressant action of cough persists for about 6 hours.

ADR: Nausea, dizziness, drowsiness, ataxia.

Dose: 10-20 mg for adults.

DIAZEPAM

Enlisted in WHO and Indian essential medicine list.

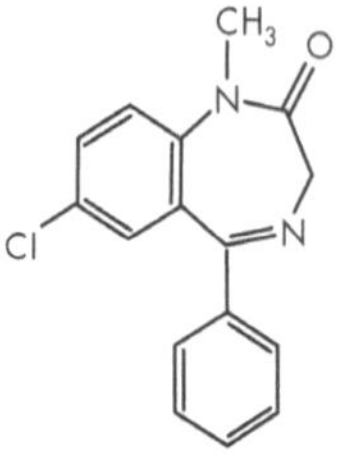

Benzodiazepine, diazepam was introduced in 1960. It is used to treat:

i. Anxiety and tension.
ii. To treat drug induced extrapyramidal symptoms and ADR of LSD.
iii. To treat acute alcohol withdrawal symptoms.
iv. As adjunct to anesthesia.
v. Anti-convulsant.
vi. As muscle relaxants.
vii. Rectal instillation for febrile convulsion.

It is absorbed rapidly and predictably after oral administration than after I.M. It produces active metabolites oxazepam. If taken with alcohol, it decreases psychomotor skills. It is cumulative.

ADR: Cleft palate, cleft lip may occur if taken in 1st trimester of pregnancy. If taken in final stage of labor it can produce low apgar score.

Blurred vision, diplopia, amnesia, slurred speech, tremor, urinary incontinence constipation, suicidal tendencies if taken more than 40-60 mg/day. Apnea, cardiac arrest may occur rarely if given I.V. route can cause pain and thrombophlebitis. Long term use of larger doses produce psychic and physical dependence.

Dose: 4-40 mg oral in adults in 2-4 divided doses or 2.5 to 10 mg at bed time. Children over 12 years of age 0.12 to 0.8 mg/kg in 3 to 4 divided doses for old and debilitated patient initial dose 2 to 2.5 mg.

I.V. and I. M. dose in adults: 2 to 5 mg for anxiety and tension for alcohol withdrawal symptoms 5- 20 mg (I.V. preferable).

Children 0.04 to 0.2 mg/kg. The I.V. should be given slowly allowing at least 1 minute for 5 mg i.e. 1 ml.

Available as 2, 5, 10 mg tab, 10 mg/2 ml inj, 2 mg/5 ml syrup.

TRADE NAME: CALMPOSE; VALIUM.

DICLOFENAC

Enlisted in Indian essential medicine list.

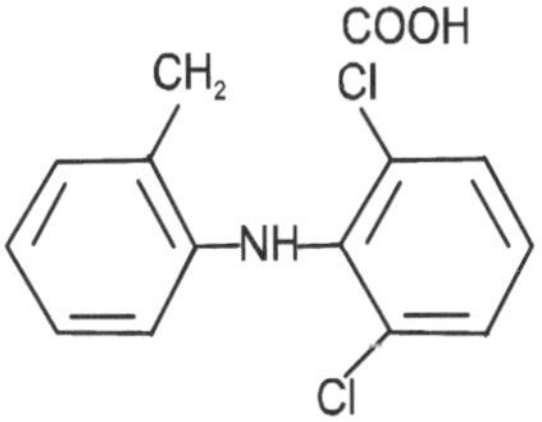

This NSAID belongs to aryl acetic acid derivative. It is PG inhibitor and to a some extent COX-2 selective. Anti-platelet function is short lasting. It reduces neutrophil chemotaxis and superoxide at inflammatory sites.

It is absorbed orally, protein bound 99%, metabolized and excreted with bile and urine. Penetrates synovial membrane and stays there for longer period so effective in joints.

ADR: Epigastric pain, nausea, headache, dizziness, rash, reversable elevation of serum amino transferase.

Therapeutic Uses: Rheumatoid, Osteoarthritis, Ankylosing spondylitis, Toothache, Bursitis, Dysmenorrhoea, Post traumatic and post operative pain.

Dose: 50 mg TDS, 75 mg deep I.M.

Available as 50 mg tab, 100 mg SR tabs, 25 mg/ml in 3 ml amp for injection, 1% topical gel, 0.1% eye drops.

TRADE NAME: VOVERAN; DICLONAC; VOLTAFLAM (It is Diclofenac Potassium).

DICYCLOMINE

Enlisted in Indian essential medicine list.

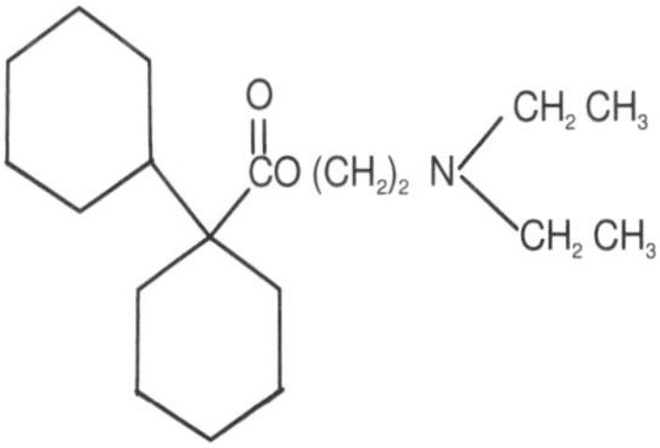

Dicyclomine is synthetic anticholinergic drug, tertiary amine used as anti-secretary, antispasmodic. It has direct smooth muscle relaxant properties.

Dose: 20 mg oral or I.M. children 5-10 mg. Not recommended below 6 months of age where it may produce atropinic toxicity. It has also been used in morning sickness, dysmenorrhoea and irritable bowel syndrome.

Available as 20 mg tab, 10 mg/ml liquid, 10 mg/ml in 2 ml injection.

TRADE NAME: CYCLOMINOL tab and liquid; CYCLOPAM Injection.

DIDANOSINE

Enlisted both in Indian and WHO's essential medicine list.

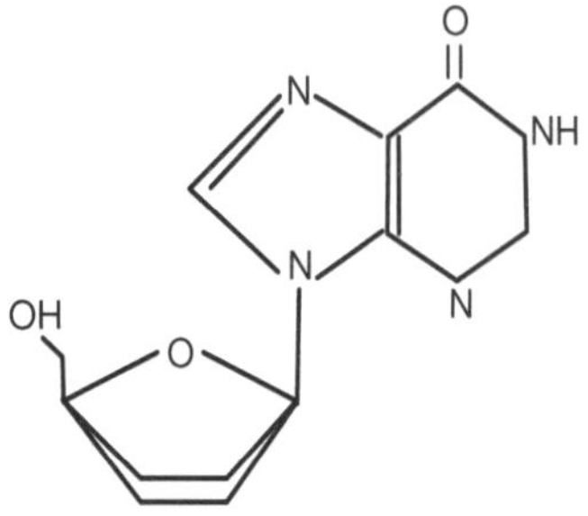

This NRTI acting against HIV-1 is synthetic analog of deoxyadenosine. When taken in empty stomach 30-40 %, is absorbed, CSF penetration is 20%. Eliminated by glomerular filtration and tubular secretion.

Available as 250, 400 mg caps; 125 and 250 mg tabs and powders.

Dose: 200 mg BD for BW below 60 kg or 125 mg BD for BW below 50 kg.

ADR: Peripheral neuropathy, pancreatitis, diarrhea, nausea, hyperuricaemia. Don't use with other neuropathic drug. It does not cause myelosuppression.

TRADE NAME: DINEX; DDRETRO.

DIETHYLCARBAMAZINE

It is enlisted both in WHO and Indian essential medicine list.

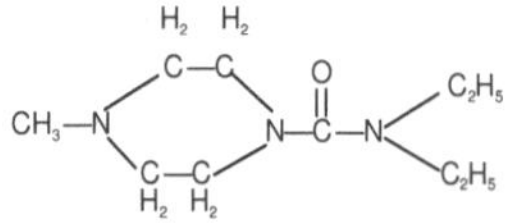

It is piperazine derivative therapeutically used for:

i. Filariasis (*W. bancrofti; W. malayi* and *Loa Loa*).
ii. Tropical eosinophilia.
iii. Onchocerciasis.
iv. Larva migrans.

It is rapidly absorbed, uniformly distributed in body except in fat metabolized in body and eliminated with urine.

ADR: Anorexia, nausea, vomiting, headache, drowsiness, allergy (fever, tachycardia, lymphadenopathy, muscle pain due to death of adult worm).

Available as 50 and 100 mg tab. and 10 mg/ml syrup.

Dose: (a) Filariasis 6-12 mg/kg × 3 weeks.

(b) Tropical eosinophilia 6-12 mg/kg 1-2 weeks.

(c) Onchocerciasis and larva migrans 2 mg/kg for 3 weeks.

TRADE NAME: HETRAZAN.

DIGOXIN

Enlisted both in WHO and Indian essential medicine list.

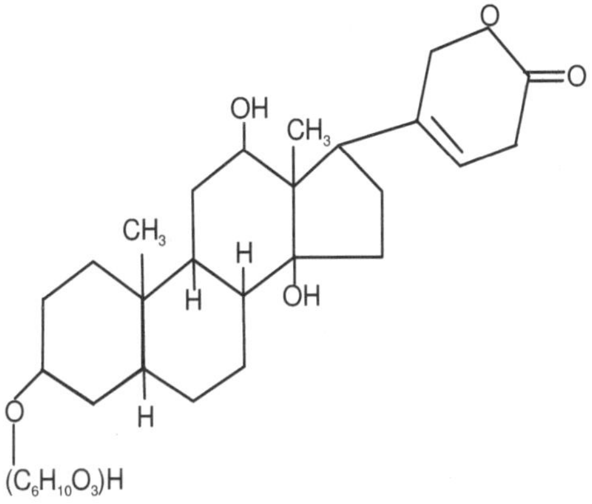

Extensively studied digitalis glycosides used both for rapid and slow digitalization. Action starts within 5-30 minutes of I.V. administration and 1-2 hours of oral administration. Its merits are: rapid, short lasting and can be given by oral or perenterally. It is excreted unchanged with urine, so dose adjustment required for renal impairment patient.

Serum therapeutic ranges from 0.5 to 2.5 ng/ml, above 3.0 ng/ml produces signs of toxicity.

Therapeutic Uses:

i. CCF.

ii. Supraventricular tachyarrythmia.

Dose: Small doses are given for elderly, hypothyroid, renal impaired patient, patient with electrolyte imbalance (hypokalaemia).

Oral (Adults): Average digitalizing dose 1-1.5 mg for rapid digitalizing 0.5 to 0.75 mg followed by 0.25 to 0.5 mg 6-8 hourly. For slow digitalization 0.125 to 0.5 mg daily.

For Children: Newborn 0.04 to 0.06 mg/kg body weight, 1 month to 2 years 0.06 to 0.08 mg/kg; over 2 years 0.4 to 0.06 mg/kg of body weight. Daily maintenance dose is 20-30% of digitalizing dose.

Intravenous Adults Dose: 0.5 to 1mg, initially 0.25 to 0.5 mg followed by 0.25 mg 4-6 hourly. For maintenance 0.125 to 0.5 mg/day.

Available as oral 0.05 mg/ml, Tabs 0.125, 0.25, 0.5 mg tablets. Injection 0.1 mg/ml, container 0.25 mg/ml in 2 ml container.
TRADE NAME: LANOXIN.

DIHYDROERGOTAMINE

Included in Indian essential medicine list.

Hydrogenation of ergotamine reduces serotonergic and α-agonistic action but increases α - blocking properly. It is weaker emetic and oxytocic. It has some anti-dopaminergic action. It is used for migraine.

Dose: 2-6 mg oral (Max 10 mg) 0.5 to1 mg I.M. or subcutaneous or I.V. repeat hourly (Max upto 3 mg).

Available as 1 mg tab, 1mg/ml injection.
TRADE NAME: DHE as tablet or MIGRANIL 1 mg/ml injection.

DILOXANIDE FUROATE

Enlisted both in WHO and Indian essential medicine list.

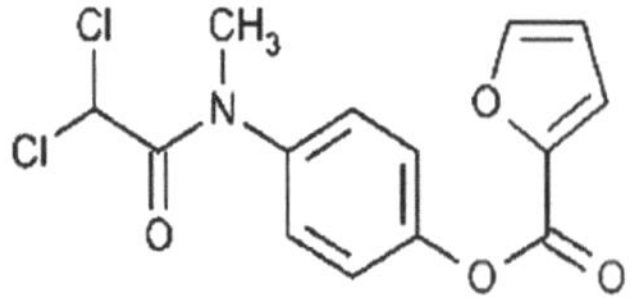

It is luminal amoebicidal; amide derivative. It directly kills trophozoites responsible for production of cysts. This ester is hydrolysed in intestine and releases diloxamide which is absorbed. Diloxamide is weaker amoebicidal than its esters. It is metabolized by glucuronidation and excreted with urine. It is poor tissue amoebicidal and a single dose produces 80-90% cure rate in intestinal amoebiasis and asymptomatic cyst passers.

Dose: 500 mg TDS × 5-10 days adults. Children 20 mg/kg/day.

Available as 500 mg tabs.
TRADE NAME: FURAMIDE.

DILTIAZEM

Enlisted in Indian essential medicine list.

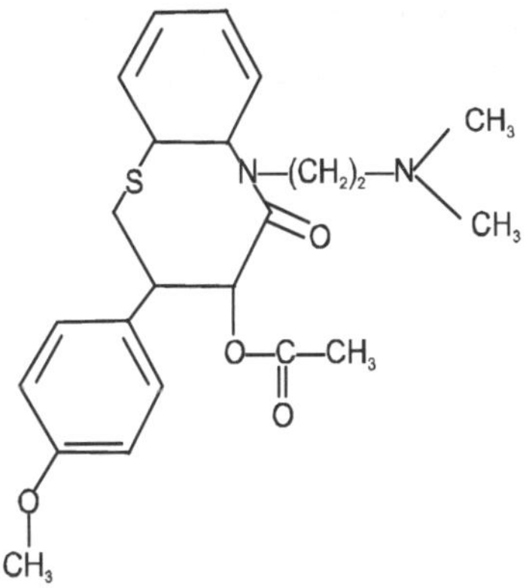

Diltiazem is hydrophilic benzothiazepine calcium channel blocker. It is less potent vasodilator than nifedipine with modest negative inotropic effects.

Therapeutically used for:

i. Angina pectoris.
ii. Hypertension.
iii. Cardiac arrhythmia (PSVT) and supraventricular arrhythmia.

ADR: Fall in BP, large doses decreases, total peripheral resistance and reflex tachycardia. It should not be given with preexisting SA and AV nodal disease and with myocardial disease. Only low dose should be given to patient receiving beta blocker.

Dose: 30-60 mg TDS.

Available as 30, 60, 90 mg (SR) tabs; 25 mg/5 ml injection. TRADE NAME: DILZEM; ANGIZEM etc.

DIMERCAPROL

WHO and Indian essential medicine enlisted drug.

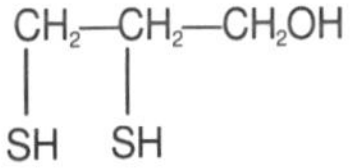

It forms stable mercaptides. The sulfydryl groups of dimercaprol remove As; Hg; Au from cellular enzymes. It is particularly useful in the treatment of acute haemorrhagic encephalitis due to massive arsenopathy. As and Au dermatitis and post arsenical jaundice. It should only be used in acute mercury poisioning not in chronic. Though it removes Pb but calcium edetate or penicillamine is preferred for their toxicity. It chelates copper but penicillin is preferred.

ADR: Pain at Injection site, paraesthesia, lacrymation, blephral spasm, asthenia, salivation, vomiting, fever and acidosis. It has a strong odour which comes to patients breath. Some of its side effects are treated by anti-histaminics. High does may cause coma and convulsion.

Dose: For As and Au poisoning 2.5 mg/kg.

QDS: 2 days, BD 3rd day, OD for 10 days.

For Hg poisoning 5 mg/kg initially; then 2.5 mg/kg OD or BD × 10 days.

Available as 100 mg/ml in peanut oil in 3 ml container.

TRADE NAME: BAL injection.

DIPHTHERIA ANTITOXIN

Enlisted both in WHO and Indian essential medicine list.

It is a sterile solution of concentrated antitoxin obtained from blood of horses hyperimmunized against diphtheria toxin.

Therapeutic Uses:

i. Diphtheria.

ii. Prophylactically in exposed, non-immunized, susceptible person, based on clinical diagnosis.

Dose: Depends upon site, extent of diphtheric membrane, degree of toxicity, duration of illness.

Usual dose: Prophylaxis 1000 to 10000 I.U. I.M., I.V. for treatment 20000-80000 I.U.

The entire dose should be given at one time as possible.

ADR: Serum sickness (urticaria, fever, pruritis, malaise and arthralgia). Skin or conjunctival test sensitivity should be done before hand.

Available as 10000 I.U./10 ml ampoule.

TRADE NAME: DIPHTHERIA ANTITOXIN.

DITHRANOL

Enlisted both in WHO and Indian essential medicine list.

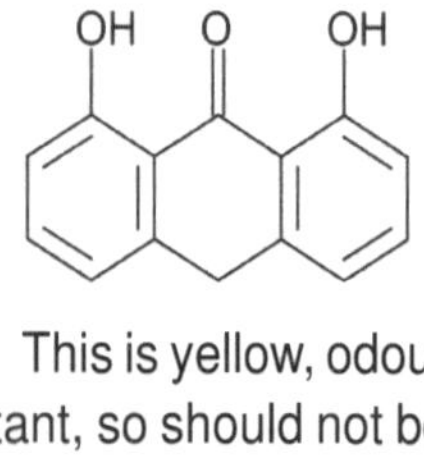

This is yellow, odourless powder, insoluble in water. It is highly irritant, so should not be applied to eyes and tender skin.

Used as 0.1 to 1% ointment; 2% paste for psoriasis, Ring worm, Chronic dermatosis, Preliminary test on a patch of skin should be done to see hypersensitivity.

TRADE NAME: ANTHRALIN.

DOBUTAMINE

Enlisted in Indian essential medicine list.

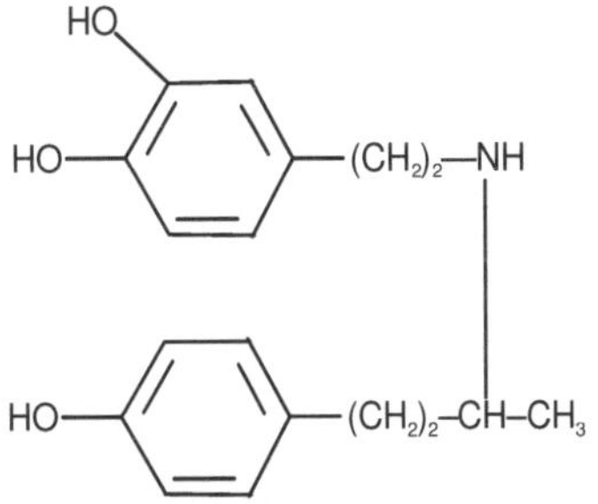

It is a derivative of Dopamine but not D_1 or D_2 agonist. It acts on α or β receptors.

Dose: 2-8 microgram/kg/min I.V. infusion. It increases C.O., force of cardiac contraction without significantly affecting heart rate and BP.

Therapeutic Uses: Pump failure as in myocardial infarction, cardiac surgery and short term management of CCF, less arrhythmogenic.

Available as 50 mg/4 ml and 250 mg/20 ml ampoules or 250 mg vial.

TRADE NAME: CRDIJET; DOBUTREX.

DOMPERIDONE

Enlisted in Indian essential medicine list.

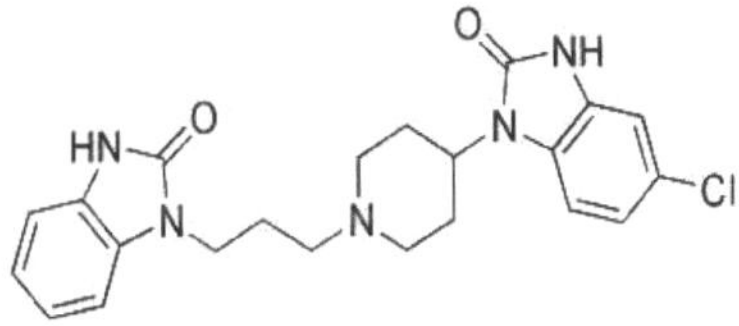

This drug is chemically related to haloperidol but pharmacologically related to metochlopramide. It is D2 receptor antagonist, orally absorbed, metabolized and excreted with urine. Crosses BBB poorly so with less extra pyramidal effect.

ADR: Dry mouth, loose motion, headache, burn, by galactorrhoea, cardiac arrhythmia (if given I.V.).

Therapeutic Uses: Low ceiling antiemetic and prokinetic administered with levodopa or Bromcriptine to counteract its dose limiting emetic action.

Dose: 10-40 mg TDS, Children 0.3 to 0.6 mg/kg.

Available as 10 mg tab, 1 mg/ml syrup.

TRADE NAME: DOMSTAL; DOMPERON.

DOPAMINE

Enlisted both in WHO and Indian essential medicine list.

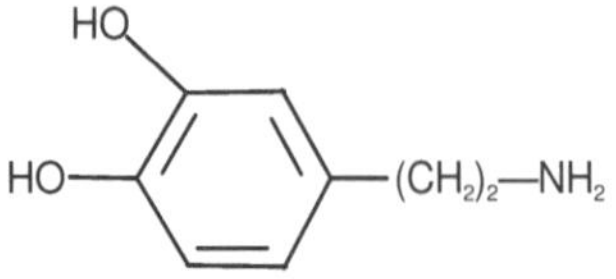

Dopamine stimulates D_1; D_2; α and β_1 receptor. The D_1 receptor present in mesenteric and renal vessels dilates to smallest I.V. infusion of Dopamine mediated through D_1 receptor as a result g.f.r and Na excretion increases. It has positive inotropic agent (due to β_1, D_1 and release of NACl). Large doses produce vasoconstriction due to α action. It does not enter CNS through BBB.

Therapeutic Uses:

i. CCF

ii. Cardiogenic and septic shock.

Dose: 0.2 – 1mg/min (Regulated by BP and urine formation).

Available as 200 mg/5 ml amp.

TRADE NAME: DOPAMINE, INTROPIN, DOPACARD.

DOXAPRAM

Indian essential medicine enlisted drug.

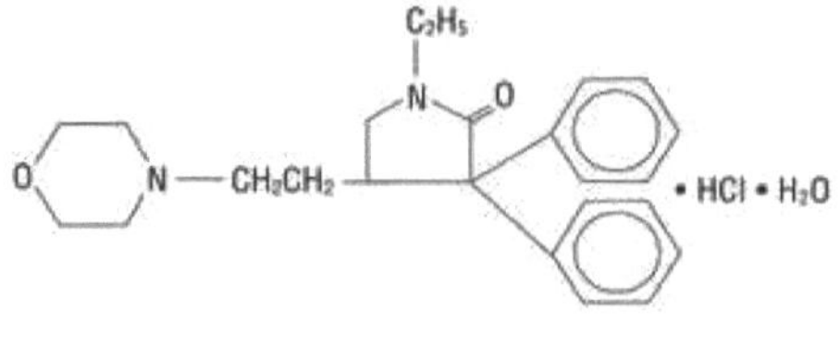

This is an analeptic (respiratory stimulants) acts by promoting excitation of central neurons. It acts at lower doses. It stimulates respiration via carotid and aortic bodies.

Therapeutic Uses: Apnoea in premature infants.

Dose: 40-80 mg I.M. or I.V., 0.5 – 2 mg/kg/hour I.V. infusion.

Available as 20 mg/ml in 5 ml amp.

TRADE NAME: CAROPRAM.

DOXORUBICIN

WHO and Indian essential medicine enlisted drug.

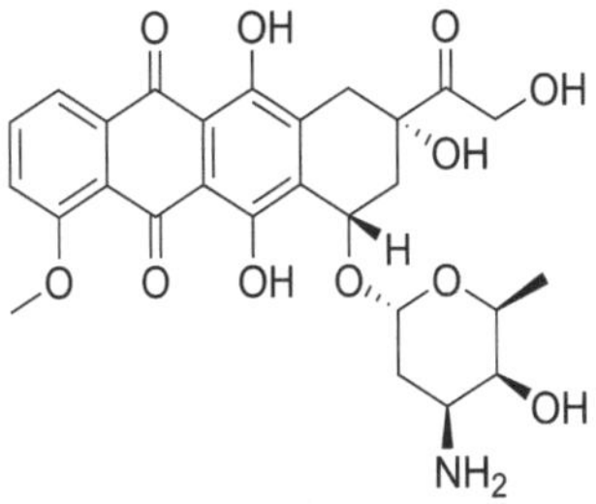

It is anthracycline antibiotic isolated from *Streptomyces pencetius var caesius,* one of the important drug to treat cancers of Breast, Endometrium, ovary, testis, thyroid, stomach, bladder, liver, lung, soft tissue cancer, neuroblastoma, Ewing's sarcoma, Osteosarcoma, Rhabdomyosarcoma.

Dose: 60-75 mg/sq mt of body surface slow I.V. every 3 weeks.

Available as 10 mg and 50 mg/vial inj.

TRADE NAME: ADRIAMYCIN; DOXORUBICIN.

DOXYCYCLINE

Enlisted both in WHO and Indian essential medicine list.

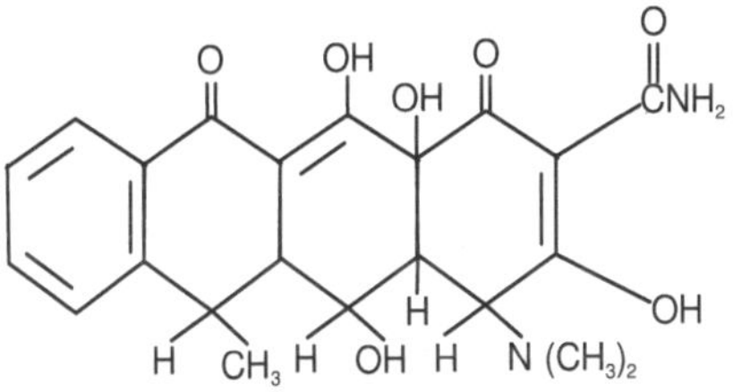

It is a tetracycline group of antibiotic (synthetic analogue of oxytetracycline). It is absorbed completely from G.I. tract. Perenteral administration is rarely done except in condition when oral administration not feasible. It is long acting t/2 15-17 hours. This tetracycline can be given to renal insufficiency patient without much increase in azotemia and its affinity for metablic ion is not that high.

Dose: Below 45 kg 100 mg BD × 2 days then 100 mg OD. Children less than 45 kg 2 mg/kg × 2 days then 1 mg /kg. I.V. dose 200 mg/day given for 1-2 infusion then 100 mg – 200 mg depending upon severity.

ADR: Like other tetracycline.

Available as Oral 50 mg/5 ml syr. Cap 50 and 100 mg. Injection powder 100-200 mg (Oral and Injections doxycycline are not available in India).

TRADE NAME: TETRADOX; DOXT.

EFAVIRENZ

WHO and Indian essential medicine enlisted drug.

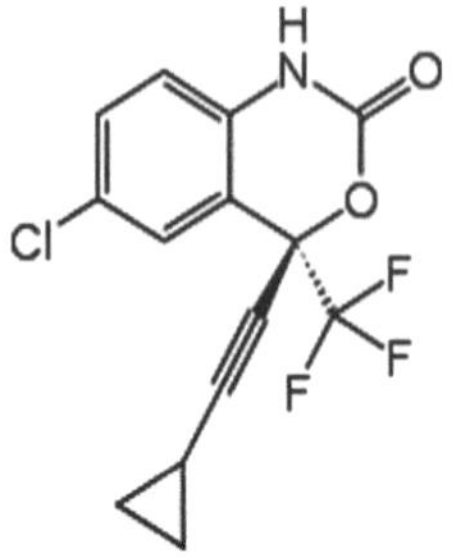

It is nonnucleoside reverse transcriptase inhibitor, used to treat HIV infection.

Dose: 600 mg daily on empty stomach because of long t/2. Bed time dosing is recommended to minimize CNS side effects. It is moderately absorbed orally. Metabolized in liver by CYP3A4 and CYP2B6 to inactive hydroxylated metabolites and remaining is eliminated with faeces. It induces and inhibits CYP3A4.

ADR: Dizziness, drowsiness, insomnia, confusion, amnesia, agitation, delusion, depression, nightmare, euphoria, i.e., CNS toxicities.

Other Toxicities: Nausea, vomiting, diarrhea, crystalluria, raises liver enzymes and serum cholesterol, foetal abnormalities if taken in pregnancy.

Available as 200 mg tab; 600 mg cap.

TRADE NAME: EVAVIR; EVIRENZ.

EFAVIRENZ + EMTRICTABINE + TENOFOVIR

EMTRICITABINE + TENOFOVIR

These combinations effective against HIV infections are enlisted in WHO's essential medicine list.

EMTRICTABINE is NRTI, fluorinated analogue of lamivudine with long t/2. Orally absorbed, not interfered by food; CSF penetration is poor.

Dose: 200 mg/daily adjust in renal insufficiency.

ADR: Headache, diarrhea, nausea, asthenia, hyperpigmentation of palm and soles.

Available as 200 mg tab.

TENOFOVIR: It is NRTI, a cyclic nucleoside phosphanate analog of adenosine. Tenofovir disopoxil fumarate is water soluble active prodrug of tenofovir. It is orally absorbed, eliminated by tubular secretion and glomerular filtration.

Dose: 300 mg QDS to take with meal. Adjust the dose in renal insufficiency.

EFAVIRENZ has been discussed earlier.

ENALAPRIL

WHO and Indian essential medicine enlisted drug.

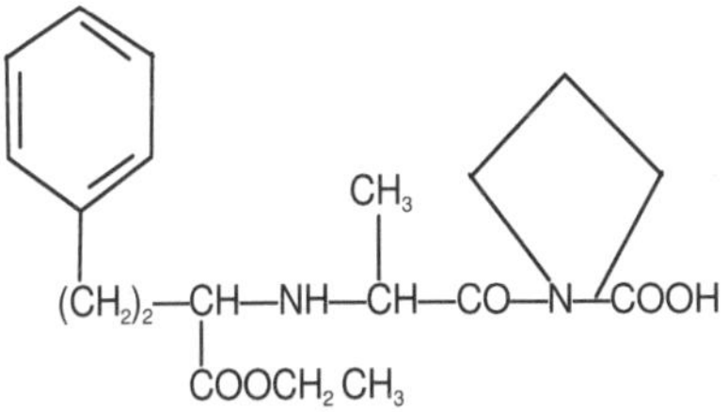

It is ACE-inhibitor. It is converted in body to enalapril at which is not orally absorbed but marketed in some countries as injectable.

It is potent, its absorption not interfered by food, slow acting, single dose therapy. Rash and loss of taste is lowers.

Therapeutic Uses:

i. Hypertension.
ii. CCF.
iii. Myocardial infarction.
iv. Diabetic and non-diabetic neuropathy.
v. Prophylactic to high cardiovascular risk subjects.
vi. Scleroderma.

ADR: i. Hypotension ii. Hyperkalemia iii. Cough iv. Rash v. Urticaria vi. Angioedema vii. Altered taste (dysgeusia) viii. Faetopathic ix. Headache, Dizziness, Nausea x. Granulocytopenia xi. Proteinuria xii. Acute real failure in a case of bilateral renal artery stenosis.

Available as 2.5, 5, 10, 20 mg tabs.

Dose: 2.5 to 20 mg depending upon severity.

TRADE NAME: ENAM; ENVAS.

EPHEDRINE

WHO enlisted essential medicine.

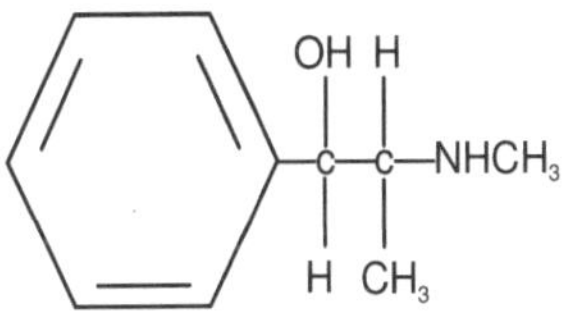

It is an alkaloid obtained from *Ephedra vulgaris*. It is indirectly acting sympathomimetic but has some direct action on α and β receptor. It produces tachyphylaxis. Long acting, crosses blood brain.

Therapeutic Uses:

i. Bronchodilatation.
ii. Nasal and ocular decongestant.
iii. Hypotensive state of anesthesia (spinal).
iv. Postural hypotension.
v. Myasthenia gravis.

ADR: Nervousness, excitability, insomnia, urinary retention in BPH patients.

Dose: 15-60 mg TDS, 3 mg/kg/day in 4-6 divided doses for children.

Available as 15, 30 mg tab, 50 mg/ml injection, 0.75% nasal drops.

TRADE NAME: EPHEDRINE HYDROCHLORIDE tab; SULFIDRIN inj., ENDERINE nasal drop.

EPINEPHRINE (ADRENALINE)

Included both in WHO and Indian essential medicine list.

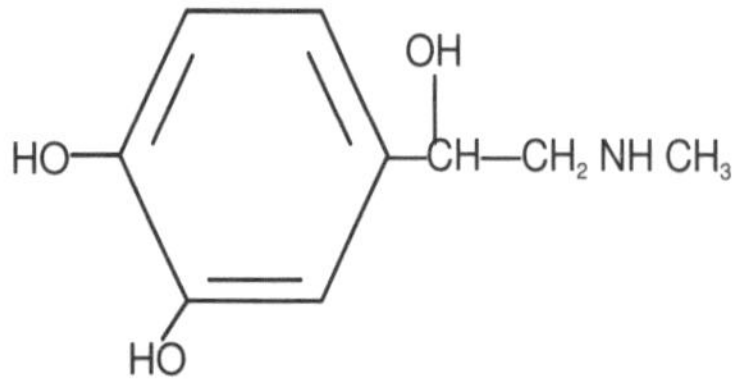

It is endogenous catecholamine. The released or exogenously Adr is partly taken up by axonal transport and metabolized by MAO and which diffuses out is acted upon by COMT. The major metabolites are excreted in urine. It is absorbed orally but are rapidly degraded by MAO and COMT of intestine and liver.

Therapeutic Uses:

i. Bronchodilatation.
ii. Allergic reactions it acts as physiologic antagonist.
iii. Glaucoma.
iv. Mydriatic.
v. Nasal decongestant.
vi. Hypotensive state.
vii. To prolonging actions of local anaesthetics.

Dose: For systemic action 0.2 to 0.5 mg S/C or I.M. Adrenaline 1 mg/ml. For vasoconstrictor 1:200,000 to 1:100000.

For primary open angle glaucoma: 2% ophthalmic solution (equivalent to 1.1% base) 1 drop BD. For ophthalmoscopy 1:1000 epinephrine soaked in wick placed in inferior cul-de-sac for 3 minutes or instilled into anterior chamber 0.2 ml 1:1000 epinephrine sulfate.

ERGOMETRINE

Enlisted in WHO's essential medicine list.

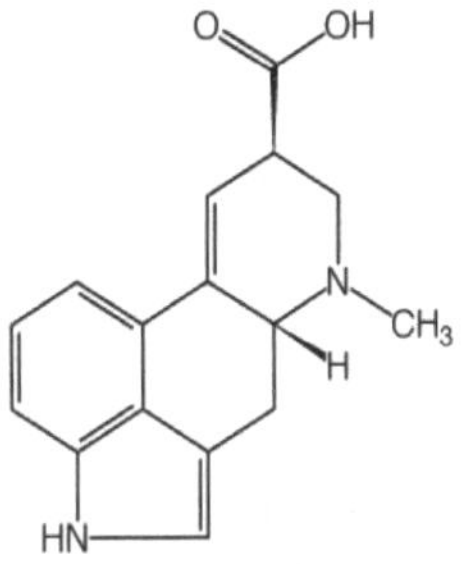

It is amine ergot alkaloid with very weak agonistic and no antagonist action on α adrenergic receptor.

Therapeutic Uses:

i. PPH
ii. To prevent uterine atony after caesarean section or forceps delivery.
iii. To induce normal involution.
iv. To diagnose variant angina.

Dose: For PPH 0.5 mg I.V.

For involution: 0.125 mg TDS × 7 days (Not in all cases).

Available as 0.25, 0.5 mg tabs; 0.5 mg/ml injection. Methylergotamine 0.125 mg tab; 0.2 mg/ml inj.

TRADE NAME: ERGOMETRINE; METHERGIN for (Methylergometrine).

ERYTHROMYCIN

Included both in WHO and Indian essential medicine list.

It is macrolide antibiotic characterized by macrocyclic lactone ring (14-16 atoms) with two deoxy sugars attached to it. It is obtained from *Streptomyces erythreus*. It is bacteriostatic in low concentration and cidal at higher concentration. It acts on 50 S ribosomal subunits of bacteria and interferes its translocation.

Therapeutic Uses:

i. Mycoplasma pneunoniae, whooping cough, chancroid as 1st choice.
ii. Pharyngitis, tonsillitis, mastoiditis, community acquired pneumonia Diphtheria, tetanus, syphilis, Gonorrhea, leptospirosis as alternative to penicillin (if hypersensitives).
iii. As 2nd choice for Campylobacter, Legionnaires pneumonia, Chlamydia trachomatosis, Penicillin resistant staph infection.

Available as:

i. **Erythromycin base** 250 mg tabs, 125 mg/5 ml. TRADE NAME: ERYSAFE.
ii. **Erythromycin stearate** 250, 500 mg tab; 100 mg/5 ml syrup; 100 mg/ml drops. TRADE NAME: ERYTHROMYCIN.
iii. **Erythromycin esteolate** (Acid stable) 250 mg; 500 mg tab; 125 mg kid tab; 125 mg/5 ml syrup, 100 mg/ml paediatric drops. TRADE NAME: ALTHROCIN.
iv. **Erythromycin ethylsuccinate** 100 mg/5 ml dry syrup; 100 mg/ml drops; 125 mg/5 ml syrup. TRADE NAME: ERYNATE.
v. **Erythromycin** 30% (Ointment). TRADE NAME: GREY OINTMENT.
vi. **Erythromycin** eye ointment 0.5%.
vii. **Erythromycin** ethyl succinate 50 mg/ml in 2 ml and 10 ml container.

Dose: I.M. 100 mg QDS, for children 150 mg/kg day in 4 divided doses for premature infants and full term newborn, 7.5 mg/kg in four divided doses.

ADR: Epigastric pain, diarrhea, hypersensitivity, hepatitis (with esteolate esters).

Interaction: QT prolongation with terfenadine, cisapride, Astemazole due to inhibition of CYP 3 A4. It raises plasma level of theophylline, valproate, carbamazepine, ergotamine and warfarin.

ESTRADIOL CYPIONATE

WHO and Indian essential medicine enlisted drug.

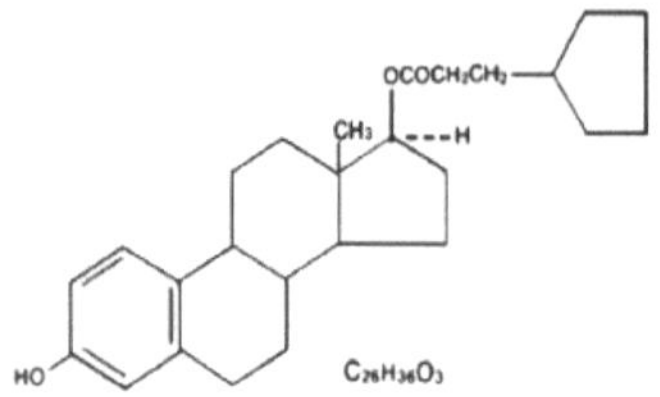

It is used for contraceptive and hormone replacement therapy in post menopausal woman.

Dose: 2.5 -10 mg I.M.

Available as 5 mg/ml in 5 ml container in cotton seed oil.

ESMOLOL

Enlisted in essential medicine list of India.

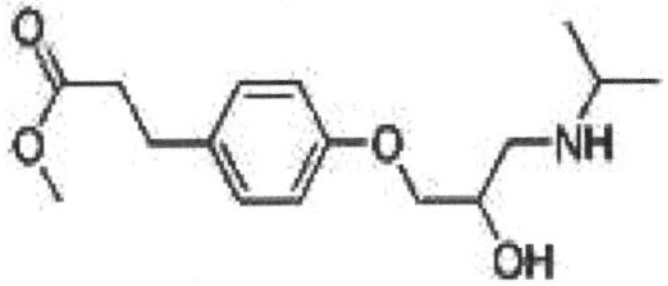

It is ultra short acting Beta blocker, devoid of partial agonisitic or membrane stabilizing actions. It is placed in class II anti-arrhythmic drug, used for quick control of ventricular rate in atrial flutter and fibrillation and supraventricular tachycardia associated with anaesthesia. It is also used to reduce BP and heart rate in cardiac surgery.

Dose: 0.5 mg/kg in 1 minute followed by 0.05 to 0.2 mg/kg per min I.V. infusion.

Available as 100 mg/10 ml and 250 mg/10 ml injection.

TRADE NAME: MINIBLOCK.

ETHAMBUTOL

WHO and Indian essential medicine enlisted drug.

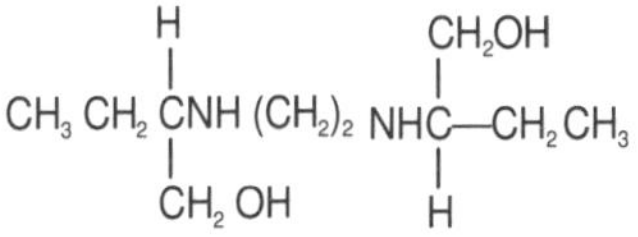

This synthetic compound has specific anti-mycobacterial effect. Orally effective, bacteriostatic, interferes mycolic acid synthesis. Resistance develops gradually due to alteration of drug target gene.

Orally administered drug is well redistributed except in meninges. Excreted by glomerular filtration and tubular excretion.

ADR: Loss of visual acuity, colour vision, optic neuritis, nausea, vomiting, rash, fever, hyperuricaemia may occur.

Dose: 15-25 mg/kg.

Available as 200, 400, 600, 800, 1 g tabs.

TRADE NAME: MYAMBUTOL; COMBUTOL.

ETHER

$C_2H_5OC_2H_5$

Enlisted in Indian essential medicine list.

This volatile liquid, used as inhalation anaesthesia, produces irritating vapour which is highly inflammable and explosive. Only minor portion is oxidized within body. 85-90% eliminated through lungs and rest through skin, urine, milk and sweat. It crosses placental barrier.

Advantages: Surgical anesthesia can be induced without preanaesthetic, has curarimimetic effect, spontaneous respiration is adequate, intermittent ether inhalation may reduce labor pain. No complicated apparatus is required, cheap.

Disadvantages: Slow onset, irritants, explosive. There may reflex inhibition of heart, nausea and vomiting during recovery and induction. Alcoholics are tolerant.

Available as: Anesthetic ether.

It is not used in developed countries because of unpleasant and inflammable nature.

Other Uses: Rubefacient, it dissolves sebaceous secretion. Preparations are:

i. Spirit of ether.
ii. Solvent ether.

ETHINYL ESTRADIOL

WHO and Indian essential medicine enlisted drug.

It is synthetic steroidal oestrogen. Used for OCP and HRT in menopausal syndrome.

Dose: 0.02-0.2 mg/day oral.

Available as 0.01, 0.05, 1 mg tab.

ADR: Suppression of libido, gynaecomastia and feminization of male organs, Epiphyseal fusion, Endometrial carcinoma, Accelerate breast cancer, risk of gall stone, hepatoma, migraine, epilepsy, endometriosis may be worsened.

TRADE NAME: LYNORAL.

ETHINYL ESTRADIOL + LEVONOR GESTREL

This combination is used in combined pill, phased pills.

In combined pill TRADE NAME: OVRAL. The dose is 50 microgram of ethinyl estradiol and 0.25 mg of levonorgestrel (a progesterone preparation). In preparation of (OVRAL-L). Ethinyl estradiol is 30 microgram and levonorgestrel is 0.15 mg.

In phased pill levonorgestrel dose is increased gradually 50, 75,125 microgram and dose of ethinyl estradiol is 30, 40, 30 microgram respectively.

TRADE NAME: TRIQUILAR 6 + 5 +10 tabs.

ETHINYL ESTRADIOL + NORETHISTERONE

This combination is enlisted both in WHO and Indian essential medicine list, used as O.C.P.

ETHIONAMIDE

WHO enlisted essential medicine.

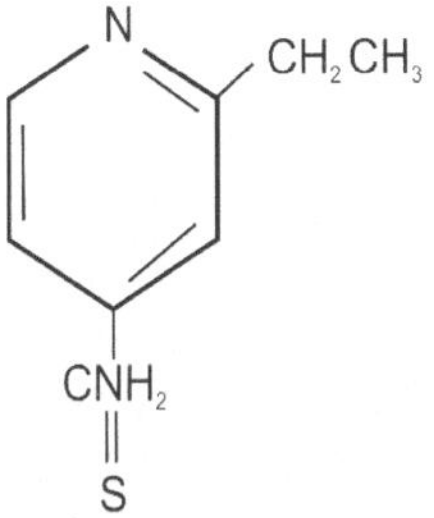

This antimicobacterial is thioamide of isonicotinic acid, but there is no cross resistance between these two agents. It is 1/10 as active as INH. It is distributed widely in body including CSF. Active both for human and bovine strain of tuberculosis. It is orally absorbed.

ADR: Anorexia, nausea, vomiting are due to CNS not due to G.I. irritation. Hepatotoxicity which recovers on drug withdrawal, peripheral neuritis and mental depression may occur.

Available as 125 and 250 mg tab.

Dose: 250 mg BD and increase it gradually fortnightly by 250 mg. Children tolerate it better. Dose 12 mg/kg in 3 divided doses.
TRADE NAME: ETHIOKOX.

ETHOSUXIMIDE

WHO enlisted essential medicine.

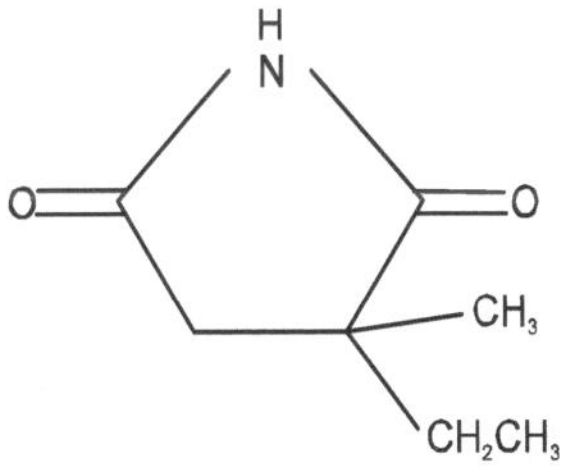

Used for absence seizure, Myoclonic spasm, Akinetic epilepsy.

ADR: G.I. disturbances, drowsiness ataxia, headache, dizziness, euphoria, hiccup, rash, behavioral changes, aplastic anaemia, thrombocytopenia, leukocytopenia, pancytopenia, SLE, parkinsonism.

Available as 250 mg caps and 250 mg/ml syrup.

Dose: 250 mg/day increased by 250 mg weekly (Above 6 years of age).

Its plasma t/2 is 30 hours for children and 60 hours for adults. Peak plasma level after single oral dose occurs in 1 to 7 hours. Serum concentration 40-100 μg/ml produces satisfactory control. TRADE NAME: ZARONTIN.

ETHYL ALCOHOL (70%) DENATURED

C_2H_5OH
Included both in WHO and Indian essential medicine list.

Aliphatic alcohols have varying degrees of antiseptic and disinfecting activity. Ethyl alcohol in widely used disinfactants for skin, better bacteriocidal action because it acts rapidly by coagulating protein. 70% alcohol reduces the surface tension of bacterial cells than undiluted alcohol which precipitating protoplasm on the periphery and retards penetration of bacteria. It is not trustable virucidal agent. Skin has to be cleansed with defatting agent prior to alcohol in surgery. It is not sporicidal, so not useful for sterilizing instruments. It is also used for cleansing, lubricants, rubifacient, and skin conditioner to cool skin (but may irritate inflamed and denuded skin). Application of emollient preparation after alcohol rub helps to alleviate dry feeling of skin. It is also used to dry to prevent "swimmers ear" and "hot weather ear" by instilling few drops of 70% alcohol which are common forms of external otitis occurs in warm weather. It is also rubbed into skin to prevent bed sore used for reducing body temperature. Injections to reduce intractable neuralgic pain. 7-10% alcohol is appetite stimulant and carminative. It is also used to treat methyl alcohol poisoning. Marketed under gerneric name.

ETHYL CHLORIDE

Enlisted in Indian essential medicine list.

It is a volatile liquid used as general anaesthetics. It is non-irritating, inflammable liquid with boiling point 12°C. Its vapour has characteristic odour. It vaporizes when sprayed on skin producing transient paralysis of cutaneous nerves. Skin should be prepared with petroleum to prevent sloughing. It causes local oedema, decreases resistance for infection and delays wound healing. Incision and drainage of abscess can only be done by these anaesthetics, as it is short lasting. It is also used as general anaesthetics which lasts 2-3 minutes and it is difficult to maintain the steady state. Muscle relaxation is poor. Other disadvantages are liver toxicity, arrhythmia.

Therefore it is used as surface anaesthesia and induction of general anaesthesia.

ETOPOSIDE

Both WHO and Indian essential medicine enlisted drug.

This is semisynthetic derivative of podophyllotoxin extract of many apple root (podophyllum peltatism) used orally and I.V. It blocks cell divison in late S and G2 phase of cell cycle. It inhibits topoisomerase II resulting DNA damage. It is highly 90% protein bound, widely distributed, except in brain.

Therapeutic Uses: Germ cell cancer, small cell and non small cell lung cancer, Hodgkin and non-Hodgkin's lymphoma, gastric cancer, breast cancer.

Dose: 50-100 mg/sq mm for 5 days.

ADR: Nausea, vomiting, hypotension, alopecia, bone marrow depression.

Available as 25, 50, 100 mg cap; 100 mg/5 ml injection.

TRADE NAME: LASTET.

FACTOR IX COMPLEX (FACTORS II; VII; IX; X)

Haemophilia B (Christmas disease) is caused by deficiency of Factor IX. Stable, dried purified preparations of Factor IX are now available commercially for intravenous use. Other factors (K dependent factors) have similar absorption properties (II; VII; X).

ADR: Viral hepatitis.

FACTOR VIII CONCENTRATE included both in WHO and Indian essential medicine list.

Deficiency of Factor VIII clotting factor produces haemophilia A. Before plasma concentrate was available it was treated with frequent infusion of plasma and blood and the large volume required for that producing hypervolemia and it has to be given fresh. Factor VIII concentrate virtually eliminated those possibilities.

It is available as precipitate or dried preparation or cryoprecipitate prepared in blood banks.

The commercial preparations are easy to handle store and administer than cryoprecipitates but commercial preparations are costly.

FERROUS SALTS

Included both in WHO and Indian essential medicine list.

Iron compounds are contraindicated in all anaemias except iron deficiency anaemia. Ferric chloride is used as throat pain. Oral is the route of choice. Ferrous compounds are better absorbed (Ferrous sulfate, Ferrous gluconate and Ferrous fumarate). It is absorbed best in between meals but it is tolerated better if taken after meal.

Elemental iron content of diferrent iron preparations differ.

For iron deficiency patient 50-100 mg of elemental iron in given. TDS is recommended for six months to replenish body iron stores. The response starts after 5-10 days and haemoglobin value starts rising after 2 weeks. Normal value comes within 2 months if there is no leakage of blood.

Perenteral iron given to those who cannot tolerate oral iron, malabsorption syndrome and apparent intolerance of oral iron is not a valid indication of iron therapy.

Some Oral Iron Preparations:

- Ferous sulfate 32% iron.
- Ferrous gluconate 12% iron.
- Ferrous fumarate 33% iron.
- Colloidal ferric hydroxide 50% iron.
- Ferrous succinate 35% iron.

Some perenteral iron preparations are:

i. Iron-dextran (TRADE NAME: INFERON 2 ml ampoules).
ii. Iron sorbitol citric acid complex (TRADE NAME: JECTOFER 1.5 ml ampoule).

ADR of Perenteral Iron Therapy: Pain, abscess, pigmentation of local site. Systematic ADR are fever, joint pain, headache, flushing headache, palpitation, dyspnoea, lymph node enlargement.

FOLIC ACID; FERROUS SALT AND FOLIC ACID; FOLINIC ACID

Folic acid in included in both WHO and Indian essential medicine list. Ferrous salt and folic acid enlisted in WHO essential medicine whereas folinic acid is WHO enlisted essential medicine.

FOLIC ACID is chemically pteroyl glutamic acid consisting of pteridine, para-aminobenzoic acid and glutamic acid. Daily requirement 0.1 mg which increases during pregnancy, lactation and of higher metabolic activity. It is used in (i) conversion of homocysteine to methonine (ii) generation of thymidylate (iii) conversion of serine to glycine (iv) purine synthesis (v) in generation of formate pool (vi) histidine metabolism.

Therapeutic Uses: Megaloblastic anaemia; pernicious anaemia. In pregnancy and lactation; anti-epileptic therapy, prophylactically in folate deficiency.

Available as 5 mg tab.

Dose: 2.5 mg/day; prophylactic < 0.5 mg/day.

TRADE NAME: FOLVITE.

Deficiency manifest as: Megaloblastic anaemia epithelial damage, glossitis, enteritis, diarrhoea, steatorrhoea, neural tube defect, spina bifida, weight loss, sterility, debility, neurological symptoms.

FOLINIC ACID: Available as 3 mg/ml injection, 15 mg tab.

Used for toxicity due to folic acid antagonist like methotrexate.
TRADE NAME: CALCIUM LEUCOVORIN; RECOVORIN.

FLUCONAZOLE

WHO and Indian essential medicine enlisted drug.

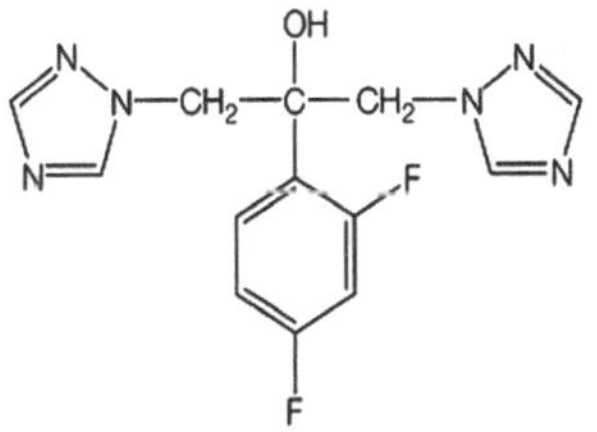

This azole (Triazole) is antifungal drug, used systematically. It is water soluble used for cryptococcal meningitis, systemic and mucosal candidiasis, coccodiodal meningitis, histoplasmosis.

94% orally absorbed, not affected by food or pH of stomach, excreted with urine.

ADR: Nausea, vomiting, adominal pain, rash, headache, elevates hepatic transaminase, should not be given to pregnant and lactating mother.

Drug Interactions: It increases plasma levels of phenytoin, astemizole, Cisapride, Cyclosporine, Warfarin, Zidovudine, Sulfonylurea.

Single 150 mg oral dose for vaginal candidiasis 150 mg/day × 2 weeks oral pharyngeal candidiasis. For cutaneous candidiasis 150 mg weekly × 4 weeks. For tinea unguium 150 mg weekly × 12 months. For disseminated candidiasis, Cryptococcal, Coccidiodal meningitis and other systemic fungal infection.

Dose: 200-400 mg/day for 4-12 weeks. Eye drops for fungal keratitis.

Available as: 50, 100, 150, 200 mg caps; 200 mg/100 ml I.V. infusion; 0.3% eye drop.
TRADE NAME: SYSCAN; FORCAN.

FLUCYTOSINE

WHO and Indian essential medicine enlisted drug.

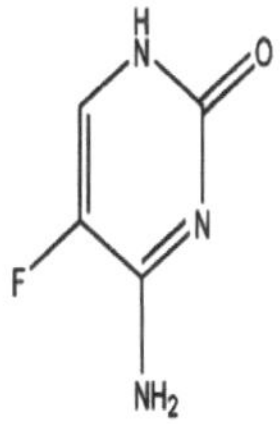

Flucytosine came out as anti-fungal drug instead of anti-cancer drug. It is water soluble fungistatic. Its spectrum is narrower than amphotericin–B. It is used in North America only. This pyrimidine antimetabolite taken up by fungal cell and converted to 5-fluorouracil and then converted to 5-fluorodeoxy uridylic acid which ultimately inhibits thymidylate synthesis. Spectrum, Cryptococcus neoformans, Torula, Chromoblastomyces, some strains of candida.

ADR: Bone marrow depression, enteritis, diarrhea, liver dysfunction. Used rarely because of toxicity.

Dose: 100-150 mg/kg/day orally.

FLUMAZENIL

Enlisted in Indian essential medicine list.

It is benzodiazepam antagonist without effect on normal subjects but competes with BZD receptor and reverses its depressive action.

It is orally absorbed but not used orally. On I.V. administration action starts in seconds and lasts 1-2 hours.

Therapeutic Uses: To reverse BZD anaesthesia and BZD overdose.

ADR: Agitation, discomfort, tearfulness, anxiety, seizure may occur. Otherwise safe.

Available as 0.1 mg/ml for I.V. injection.

FLUORESCEIN

Included in WHO and Indian essential medicine list.

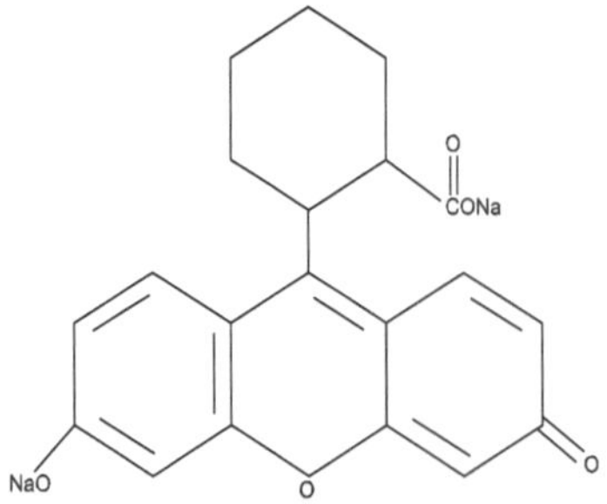

This indicator dye appears yellow green in normal tear and bright green in alkaline medium like aqueous humor.

Therapeutic Uses:

i. Topically in fitting hard contact lens.
ii. To locate the site of wound leak after cataract surgery.
iii. To test lacrimal patency.

Given I.V. for:

i. Retinal photography.
ii. Carotid artery occlusion as for irrigating eye after injury or to detoxify aniline dye of pencil causing eye injury.

ADR: Contamination of fluorescein for local use, nausea, vomiting may occur after I.V. administration.

Dose: 1 drop of 2% solution for topical application. For tonometry 0.25% solution. To detect epithelial defect 0.5-2%, for lacrimal patency 2% solution: As antidote of aniline dye 2% solution.

I.V. for adults 500 mcg (10 ml of 5% solution or 5 ml of 10% solution).

5- FLUOROURACIL (5 FU)

Enlisted both in WHO and Indian essential medicine list.

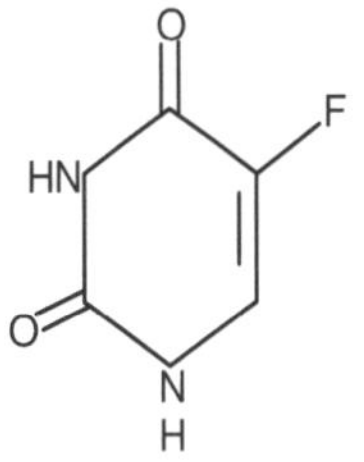

5 FU is pyrimidine antagonist is a prodrug requiring activation, produces anti-cancer effect by acting both on DNA and RNA.

Therapeutic Uses: Colorectal cancer and solid tumors (Breast, stomach, pancreas, oesophagus, liver, head, neck).

ADR: Nausea, Mucositis, Diarrhoea, Bone marrow depression, Neurotoxicity.

Dose: 15 mg/kg/day, I.V. × 5 days.

Or 1 gm orally on alternate day.

Available as 250 mg cap, 250 mg/5 ml, for I.V. or 1% topical solution.

TRADE NAME: FLURACIL; FIVE FLURO.

FLUOXETINE

Included both in WHO and Indian essential medicine list.

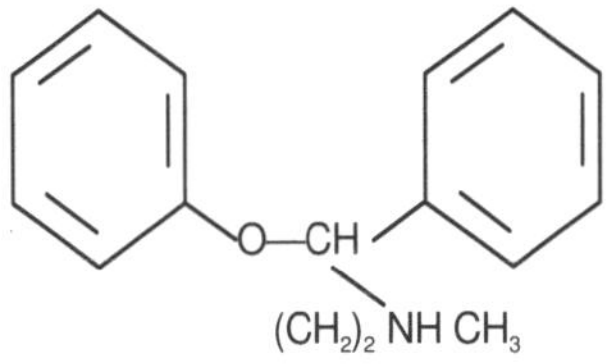

It is selective serotonin receptor reuptake inhibitors SSRI. Bicyclic compound, plasma t/2 2 days. Activated to active metabolite. Used for depression, OCD.

ADR: Agitation, Dermatological reaction.

Dose: 20-50 mg/day.

Available as: 20 mg cap, 20 mg/5 ml suspension.

TRADE NAME: FLUDAL; FLUNIL.

FLUPHENAZINE

WHO enlisted essential medicine.

It is high potency phenothiazines with piperazine side chain with minimal autonomic side effects. Hypotension, sedation and lowering seizure threshold is less extrapyramidal effect is marked. Fluphenazine decanoate is depot preparation.

Available as 1 mg tab, 0.5 mg/ml elixir and as depot preparation as mentioned.

TRADE NAME: ATATENSOL.

FLUTAMIDE

Enlisted in Indian essential medicine list.

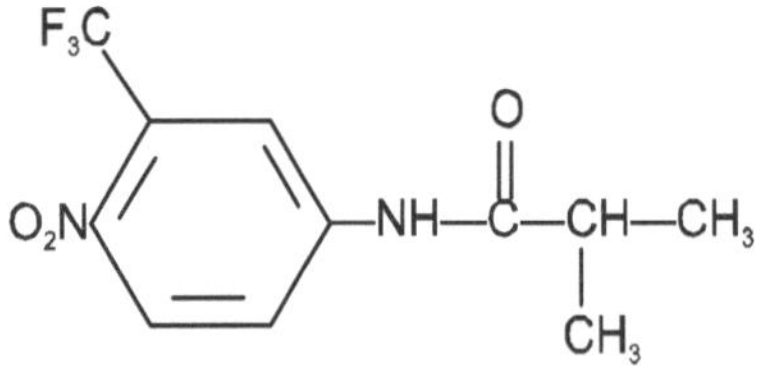

Non-steroidal drug with anti androgenic effects 2-hydroxyflutamide is its active metabolite competitively blocks androgen receptor.

Therapeutic Use: Metastatic prostatic cancer along with OCP to treat female hirsutism.

ADR: Gynaecomastia, Breast tenderness, liver damage.

Dose: 250 mg TDS.

Available as 250 mg tab.

TRADE NAME: PROSTAMID; FLUTIDE.

FORMALDEHYDE

H—CH—O

Enlisted in Indian essential medicine list.

It is gas at room temperature, used as fumigant 34% w/w. 1:200 is disinfectant. It is extremely irritant.

Therapeutic Uses:

i. Disinfection of surgical gloves and instruments 2-5%. For disinfecting excreta sputum 10%.
ii. To dress septic root canal.
iii. For removal of warts of palms and soles 3%.
iv. Preservative of pathological specimens (4%).
v. Gaseous formaldehyde for sterilization.

FRAMYCETIN SULFATE

Enlisted in Indian essential medicine list.

This is antibiotic, topically used on eye, skin and ear. Systematically it is very toxic.

Available as 1% skin cream, 0.5% eye drops or ointment.

It is obtained from *S. Levendulare.*

TRADE NAME: SOFRAMYCIN.

FRESH FROZEN PLASMA

Enlisted in Indian essential medicine list.

It contains all blood proteins (Albumin, globulin and fibrinogen) obtained from a single donor. When other suitable derivatives are not available or when multiple clothing factors deficiency is believed to be the cause of the disease, it is used. It is also given for hypovolemia, haemoconecentration of burn shock and to maintain colloidal oncotic pressure. Bleeding due to anticoagulant therapy can be controlled.

FURAZOLIDINE

Enlisted in Indian essential medicine list.

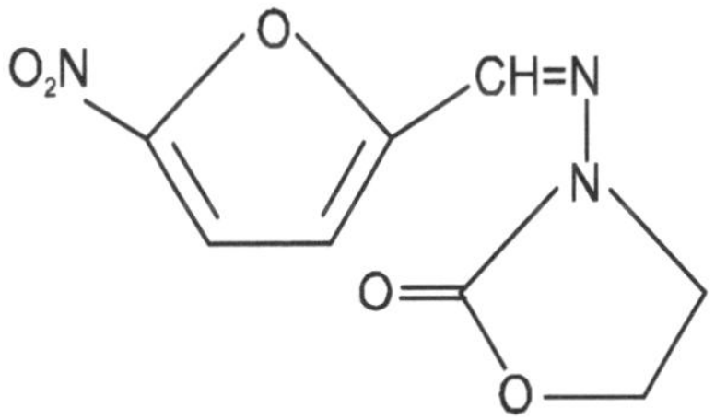

Nitrofuran compound. Active against Salmomella, Shigella, Giardia, Trichomonas.

Dose: 100 mg TDS × 5-7 days for giardia. Also used for bacterial enteritis, food poisoning, bacillary dysentery. It is partly orally absorbed and excreted with urine (so it turns orange).

ADR: Nausea, Headache, Dizziness, Antabuse like action.

Available as 100 mg tab, 25 mg/5 ml syrup.

TRADE NAME: FUROXONE.

FUROSEMIDE

Enlisted both in WHO and Indian essential medicine list.

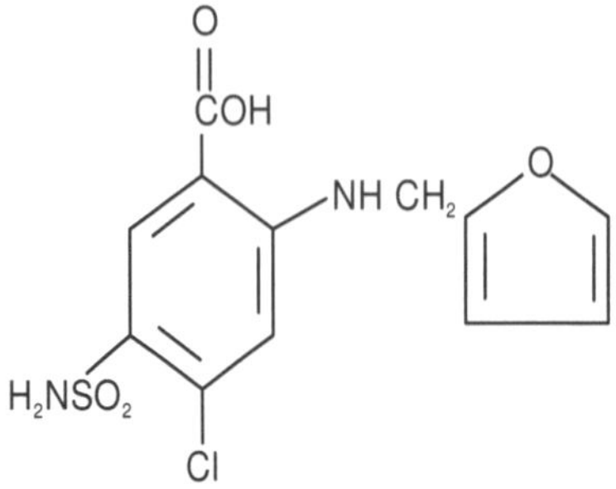

This is high ceiling (Loop diuretic). Inhibits $Na^+ K^+2Cl^-$ co-transport. Its diuretic response increases on increasing the dose (may go upto 10L).

Its onset is 2-5 min on I.V., 10-20 min on I.M. 20-40 minutes after oral administration.

It is orally absorbed, low lipid soluble, highly protein bound. Conjugated to glucuronic acid and mainly excreted unchanged by glomerular filtration and tubular secretion.

Dose: 20-80 mg once daily in morning upto 200 mg 6 hourly.

Available as 40 mg tab, 20 mg/2 ml injection and also in high dose 500 mg tab; 250 mg/125 ml injection and also in high dose 500 mg tab; 250 mg/125 ml injection.

Therapeutic Uses: Oedema, acute pulmonary oedema following myocardial infarction, cerebral oedema, hypertension, along with blood transfusion, hypercalcaemia, forced diuresis in poisoning.
TRADE NAME: LASIX.

GAMMA BENZENE HEXACHLORIDE

Indian essential medicine enlisted drug.

This broad spectrum insecticide kills lice and mites by penetrating their chitinous cover and affecting nervous system.

Therapeutic Uses: Lice, scabies both of them can develop resistance to it, which can be decreased by combining it with Benzyl benzoate.

Available as 1% ointment and lotion.

For scabies the lotion or ointment is applied over the body below neck, kept for 12-24 hours and bath is taken after. May be repeated after 1 week. For pediculosis apply to hair, leave for 12-24 hours and then wash off. May be repeated after one week if required.

It may be absorbed via skin to produce systemic toxicity viz, vertigo, convulsion, CNS stimulation cardiac arrhythmia, the systematically absorbed is deposited in fat. It is inducer of cytochrome enzymes. Better to avoid it in young children and pregnant woman.

TRADE NAME: GAB, GABADERM Lot.

GEMCITABINE

Enlisted in Indian essential medicine list.

This is anti-cancer drug used for pancreatic cancer, non small cell lung cancer, bladder cancer, non-Hodgkin's lymphoma.

It is pyrimidine antagonist.

ADR: Nausea, vomiting, diarrhoea, myelosuppression.

Dose: 1000 mg/sq mm body surface I.V. weekly for seven weeks followed by rest of 1 week.

GENTAMICIN

Included both in WHO and Indian essential medicine list.

It is systemic aminoglycoside, obtained from *Micromonospora purpurae.* The main differences from streptomycin. :

More potent, spectrum includes *P. S aeruginosa, Proteus, E.coli, Klebsiella, Enterobacter, Serratia* but not effective against *M. tuberculosis, Strepto pyogenes* and pnenmonia. Its neprotoxicily is more.

Therapeutic Uses: It is cheaper. Its use should be restricted for severe gram negative infection.

i. RTI (critically ill and with impaired host defense, post operative pneumonia.
ii. Infection by Pseudomonas, Proteus, Klebsiella, UTI, Burn, Lung abscess, Osteomyelitis, Otitis media, Septicemia.
iii. Meningitis.
iv. Endocarditis.

Dose: 3-5 mg/kg/day either single or 8 hourly divided doses with creatinine clearance of 100 ml/min.

Available as 20, 60, 80, 240 mg/vial 0.3%, Ear drop, 0.1% skin ointment.

TRADE NAME: GARAMYCIN; GENTICYN; SEPTOPAL.

(It is Gentamicin polymethyl methacrylate with acrylic bead impregnated with 7.5 mg of gentamicin sulfate used for osteomyelitis).

Adjustment of dose with renal insufficiency

Creatinine clearance ml/min	% of dose
70	70%
50	50%
30	30%
10-30%	60% on alternate day
< 10	40% on alternate day

GENTIAN VIOLET

Enlisted in essential medicine list of both the WHO and India.

This rosanaline dye is an antiseptic, active against gram-positive bacteria, fungi but without effect on gram negative and mycobacterium. 0.5-1% aqueous solution is used to treat furunculosis, bed sores, chronic ulcer, infected eczema, thrush, ring worm. It stains the part, so not very popular.

GLIBENCLAMIDE

WHO and Indian essential medicine enlisted drug.

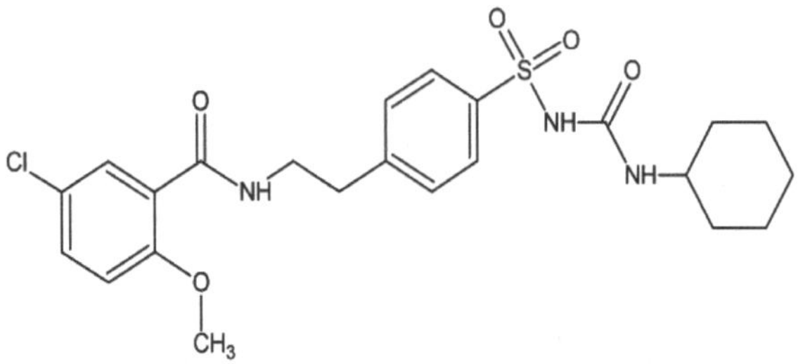

It is 2nd generation sulfonylurea used to treat type II diabetes mellitus. It acts on sulfonylurea urea receptor over β cells of pancreas to release insulin.

It is orally absorbed, protein bound, metabolized in liver, slow acting. Incidence of hypoglycemia is more. Plasma t/2 4-6 hours. Action lasts 18-24 hours.

Dose: 5-15 mg OD to BD.

Available as 2.5 and 5 mg tab.

TRADE NAME: DAONIL; EUGLUCON.

GLUCAGON

Enlisted in Indian essential medicine list.

Glucagon is single chain polypeptide secreted by α cells of pancreas, which increases blood glucose level.

Available as1 mg inj.

Since it is protein is natural, not absorbed orally t/2, 3-6 min. Broken down in liver, kidney, plasma and other tissues.

Therapeutic Uses:

i. Hypoglycaemia.
ii. As inotropic agent in cardiogenic shock.
iii. To diagnose pheochromocytoma.

GLUCOSE

Enlisted both in WHO and Indian essential medicine list.

Therapeutic Uses:

i. Diabetic hypoglycaemia.
ii. Hyperkalaemia.
iii. Perenteral therapy if oral feeding not feasible. It is generally administered I.V. as 5% which is almost isotonic to blood. Provides 170 cal/L. 10% Dextrose is used to provide more energy.
iv. 20 and 50% Dextrose is used to treat.
   a. Cerebral oedema.
   b. Sclerosing agent.
   c. To shift K^+ into the cell.

Subcutaneous administration is not desirable because of its irritant nature.

GLUCOSE WITH SODIUM CHLORIDE

It is the solution of Dextose 5% with NaCl 0.11% to 0.45% and is preferred for I.V. therapy, where water loss is more to Na loss.

ADR: Hyperglycaemia, Glycosuria, Diuresis. It clumps and haemolyzes RBC (Dextrose) which can be avoided using 5% dextrose with 0.2% to 0.9% NaCl.

GLUTARALDEHYDE

Enlisted in WHO and Indian essential medicine list.

It has wide range of biocidal activity, rapidly sporicidal and tuberculocidal. A 2% solution buffered with 0.3% sodium carbonate to a pH of 7.5 to 8.5 is useful for disinfection and sterilization of endoscopy instrument, rubber gloves. It is costly and lacks stability (Activity is lost within 2 weeks). Used for treatment of warts and hyperhidrosis.

GLYCERIN

Enlisted in Indian essential medicine list.

$CH_2\,OH$
|
$CH\,OH$
|
$CH_2\,OH$

It is used as:

i Pharyngeal demulcent to treat cough.
ii Orally active osmotic diuretic. Dose 0.5 – 1.5 g/ kg as 50-75% solution (lemon juice may be added to flavor it and to increase palatability) with crushed ice and drinking through straw), used for reducing intraocular and intracranial tension. Available as 50 and 70% solution.
iii. It is applied on dry skin and cracks 5% acting as emollient.

iv. Applied to anal canal as suppository. Undiluted glycerin is clear, sweet, viscous liquid with dehydrating property. It produces warm sensation and irritates mucous membrane.

GLYCERYL TRINITRATE

WHO and Indian essential medicine list enlisted drug.

Glyceryl trinitrate (GTN) is anti-anginal drug, rapidly denitrated enzymatically in smooth muscle cells to release reactive free radical nitric oxide (NO) which activates cytosolic cGMP causing dephosphorylation of myosine light chain kinase (MLCK). Reduced availability of MLCK relaxes smooth muscles.

ADR: Headache, flushing, weakness, sweating, palpitation, dizziness, fainting (Relieves on lying down), methemolgobinemia in increased doses, rashes rarely.

GTN is explosive volatile liquid adsorbed in inert matrix of table to make it non-explosive, stored in tightly closed glass container. It is given sublingually to abort ischaemic attack and then crushed by teeth to spread over mucous membrane. Action starts within 1-2 minutes. It can be given as sublingual spray. Metabolised by liver (so large oral dose required) can be given I.V. unstable angina, LVF with M.I., coronary spasm.

Dose: 5-20 microgram/minute I.V.

Available as 0.5 mg tab, 2.4 and 6.4 controlled release tab, skin patch or spray.

TRADE NAME: ANGISED; GTN SPRAY; NITROCONTIN; NITRODERM TTS PATCH; MROVIN.

Therapeutic Uses:

i. Angina pectoris.
ii. Acute coronary syndrome.
iii. MI.
iv. CCF and LVF.
v. Biliary colic.
vi. Esophageal spasm.
vii. Cyanide poisoning.

GRISEOFULVIN

WHO and Indian essential medicine enlisted drug.

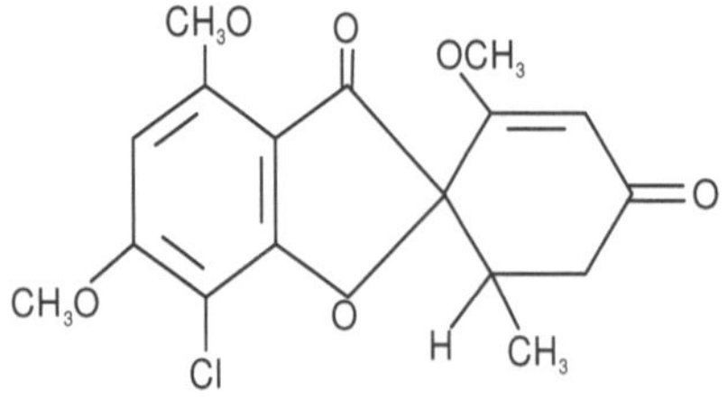

Griseofulvin is chemically heterocyclic benzfuran, fungistatic antibiotic, obtained from *Penicillium griseofulvum.* It interferes with mitosis of multinucleated hyphae.

It is low water soluble so its absorption is irregular from G.I.T. Its absorption increases after taking it with fatty meal and if the drug is microfined. It is deposited on skin, keratin and retained in tinea infected cells. Duration of treatment depends upon site of infection and turnover of keratin. Metabolized by methylation and excreted with urine.

ADR: Headache, peripheral neuritis, rash, photoallergy, leucopenia, albuminuria.

Therapeutic Uses: Dermatophytosis, Athelets food.

Available as 125 and 250 mg F.P.

Doses: 125 – 250 mg QDS with meals. Duration:

Skin of body: 3 weeks.

Palm and sole: 4-6 weeks.

Finger nails: 4-6 months.

Toe nails: 8-12 months.

Drug Interaction:

i. Induces metabolism of warfarin.
ii. Phenobarbitone induces metabolism and decreases its absorption causing therapeutic failure.
iii. Intolerance to alcohol.

HAEMOPHILUS INFLUENZAE (B) VACCINE (HIB)

WHO enlisted essential medicine list.

This bacterial vaccine contains medium oligosaccharide of H. influenzae type (b)10 microgram conjugated with non-toxic protein 25 microgram of CRM mutant C. diphtheria toxin along with aluminium hydroxide. It is given in 2-6 months of age of infants to protect against H. influenzae meningitis.

Doses: 3 doses 0.5 ml I.M. starting at 2-6 months at 8 weeks gaps. If started at 7-11 months 2 doses, one year of age required single dose.

Available as 0.5 and 5 ml vial.

TRADE NAME: HIB TITER, VAXEM HIB.

HALOPERIDOL

WHO and Indian essential medicine enlisted drug.

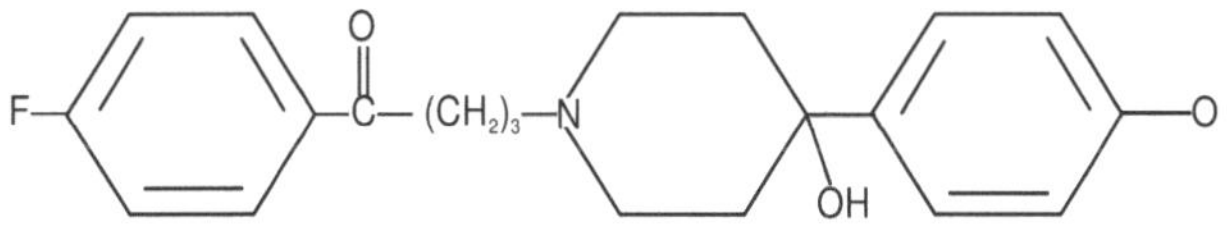

This antipsychotic drug is butyrophenone derivative. The better part of this drug is that it has less autonomic effect, less epileptogenic, no weight gain.

Therapeutic Uses:

i. Schizophrenia.
ii. Huntington's disease.
iii. Gilles de la Tourette's syndrome.

Available as 2.5, 5, 10, 20 mg tab; 2 mg/ml vial 5 mg/ml injection.

Dose: 2-20 mg/day.

TRADE NAME: SERENACE; HALOPIDOL; SENORM.

HALOTHANE

WHO and Indian essential medicine enlisted drug.

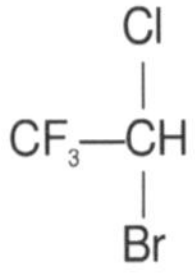

It is non-inflammable, halogenated, hydrocarbon, anaesthetic agent, volatile, liquid with sweet odour. It is non-irritants. 2-4% is required for induction, 0.5 to 1% for maintenance. Muscle relaxant and analgesic power is poor. It potentiates competitive muscle relaxants. It decreases myocardial contractility, cardiac output is reduced. It decreases sympathetic activity and augments vagal tone, sensitizes heart to ach. arrhythmia may occur. It depresses respiratory centre (so it is reprod and shallow), ventilatory support with added oxygen is required. It decreases pharyngeal and laryngeal reflexes; decreases urine formation. Hepatitis may occur. May produce malignant hyperthermia. Halothane entering blood is metabolized in liver, rest is exhaled. Its recovery is smooth and quick, shivering may occur.

Its deficiency of muscle relaxant and analgesia is compensated by concomitant use of N_2O and neuromuscular blockade.

HEPARIN SODIUM

Both WHO and Indian essential medicine enlisted drug.

Heparin is sulfated mucopolysaccharides normally present in body in mast cells; physiological role not known may be playing some role in anaphylactic shock. It is used perenterally as anticoagulants when rapid effect is desired. It is strongest naturally occurring acid, the electronegative change binds to electropositive charges of proteins of clothing mechanism and reversibly inactivates them. It does not cross B.B.B. and placenta.

Therapeutic Uses:

i. Extracorporeal circulation in open heart surgery and renal haemodialysis.
ii. Deep vein thrombosis.
iii. Pulmonary infarction.
iv. Mixed with donor blood.

ADR: Bleeding, Thrombocytopenia, Alopecia, Osteoporosis, Hypersensitivity.

Contraindication: Thrombocytopenia, bleeding disorder, severe hypertension (Risk of cerebral haemorrhage), subacute bacterial endocarditis, ocular and neurosurgery or lumbar puncture, cirrhosis, renal failure with aspirin and anti-platelet drugs.

Available as 1000-5000 I.U./ml in 5 ml vial for injection.

TRADE NAME: BEPARINE; HEPARIN SOD; PROTAMINE SULFATE IS HEPARIN ANTAGONIST.

HEPATITIS A AND HEPATITIS B VACCINES

Hepatitis A vaccine is included in WHO's essential medicine list whereas Hepatitis B vaccine is included both in WHO and Indian essential medicine list.

Hepatitis A Vaccine: Human diploid cell culture grown hepatitis virus is inactivated by formaldehyde. 0.5 ml I.M. injection is given I.M. in deltoid muscle and booster dose by same route after 6 months is recommended.

Available as 0.5 ml of prefilled syringe or 0.5 ml of injection.

TRADE NAME: AVAXIM, HAVRIX.

Hepatitis B Vaccine: It is prepared in yeast cells by recombinant technique and the contain is adsorbed in aluminium hydroxide. A 20 microgram/1ml suspension is prepared and given in 0,1,6 months. Children below 10 years is given 0.5 ml. It is included in universal immunization (specially indicated for surgeons, dentist, blood bank personal, laboratory tecnicians, haemodialysis patient, hemophiliacs, drug addicts).

ADR: Fever, malaise, local soreness, vomiting may occur.

HOMATROPINE

It is Indian essential medicine enlisted drug.

This semi-synthetic derivative anti-cholinergic drug is used for:

Mydriatic and cycloplegic (2% to 5%) solution at 10 minutes interval is topically instilled for refraction, testing and uveitis.

Homatropine methyl bromide (2.5 – 10 mg QDS for adults and 3.6 mg QDS in children) used as anti-spasmodic.

ADRs are like other anti-cholinergic drugs.

HYDRALAZINE

WHO enlisted essential medicine.

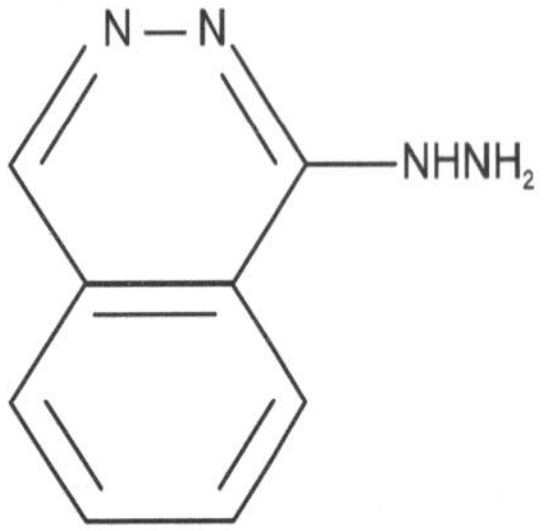

Hydralazine lowers BP by relaxing arteriolar smooth muscles with little effect on capacitance vessels, which evokes the reflex compensatory mechanism causing tachycardia; rise in cardiac output, renin release, Na and H_2O retention producing hyperdyamic circulatory state and angina may be precipitated. Tolerance to hypotension action develops which can be blocked by diuretics and beta blockers. Its smooth muscle relaxants action is probably due to nitric oxide.

It is orally absorbed, first pass metabolism in liver acetylated (some are slow and some are fast acetylators) and excreted with urine.

Therapeutic Uses: Hypertension not controlled by 1st line drug and in patient with renal impairment. Contraindicated in older patient and IHD patients safe in pregnancy, used for CCF also.

Dose: 25-50 mg OD to TDS.

Available as 25 mg tab.

TRADE NAME: NEPRESOL.

HYDROCHLOROTHIAZIDE

Enlisted both in WHO and Indian essential medicine list.

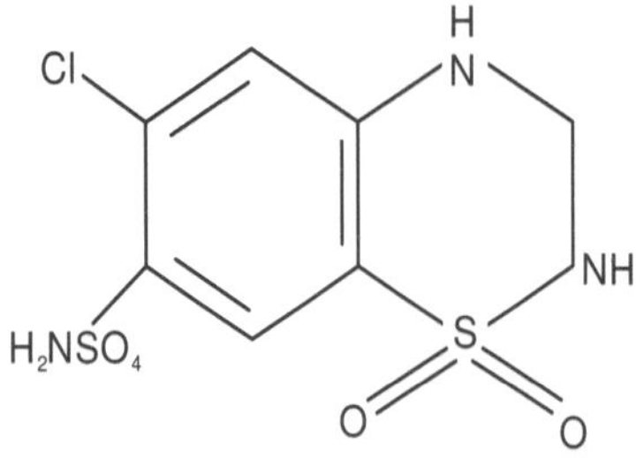

This medium efficiency diuretic inhibits Na^{+}-Cl^{-} symports.
Used for:

i. Oedema.
ii. Hypertension.
iii. Diabetes insipidus.
iv. Hypercalciuria.

Complications

Hypokalemia, acute saline depletion, hyponatraemia, nausea, vomiting, diarrhoea, headache, giddiness weak-nes, paraesthesia, hearing loss, rash, photosensitization, hyperuricemia hyperglycemia, hyperlipidemia, hypercalcaemia, Mg-depletion. May precipitate renal insufficiency, hepatic coma in cirrhotic may be precipitated. Do not use in toxemia of pregnancy because it may compromise circulation and cause foetal death.

Available as: 12.5; 25; 50 mg tab.

Dose : 12.5 to 100 mg/day.

Interaction: Potentiates anti-hypertensives; Hypokalemia induces digitalis toxicity; oto and nephrotoxic with aminoglycosides; may cause thrombocytopenia with co-trimoxazole; serum lithium level rises indomethacin blunts its action.

TRADE NAME: AQUAZIDE; HYDRIDE.

HYDROCORTISONE

Enlisted in WHO essential medicine list.

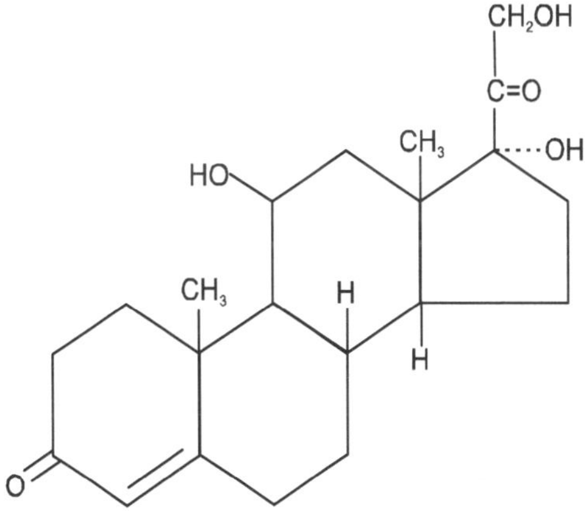

It is rapid and short acting corticosteroid has glucocorticoids and significant mineralocorticoid action. It can be given orally or I.V. for acute and chronic adrenocortical insufficiency, including adrenogenital syndrome, shock, status asthmaticus. Its use as anti-inflammatory action is limited because of mineralocorticoid action. It is also used topically and as enema (for ulcerative colitis).

Preparations available:

Oral: Hydrocortisone, hydrocortisone cytrionate.

Dose: 10-20 mg daily. For adrenocortical insufficiency for life threatening disease upto 60-120 mg.

Intravenous (Hydrocortisone as sodium phosphate sodium succinate).

Dose: 100-500 mg.

Intramuscular 100-250 mg (maximum upto 1 gm).

Topical (Hydrocortisone, hydrocortisone acetate) applied TD or QD.

Rectal (Hydrocortisone enema) one enema every 21 days.

Hydrocortisone sodium succinate is enlisted in Indian essential drug list and is used for same purposes.

TRADE NAME: EFCORLIN (100 mg/2 ml as hemisuccinate).

ENTOFOAM (10% cream or enema for distal ulcerative colitis patient).

HYDROGEN PEROXIDE (H_2O_2)

Included in Indian essential medicine list.

H_2O_2: Hydrogen peroxide when comes in contact with enzyme found in blood and most of the tissues, are rapidly decomposed to water and oxygen and the liberated oxygen has bacteriocidal effect till is liberated. It looses masses by mechanical effect of liberated oxygen. It may be used as gargle, mouth wash and vaginal douche. 3% is used to remove wax of ear. It should not be applied in close body cavities and abscess from which gas has no free egress.

There is report of hemiplegia on its application on pleural cavities likely due to the passage of the gas into vascular system producing embolism.

HYDROXYCOBALAMINE

WHO enlisted essential medicine list. Discussed with Vit B_{12}.

HYDROX ETHYL STARCH (HES)

Enlisted in Indian essential medicine list.

This plasma expander is a complex mixture of ethoxylated amilopectin of various sizes; mol weight 10000 to million average 4.5 lac. 6% of HES has colloidal properties of that of albumin smaller m.w. are rapidly excreted by kidney; larger molecules are slowly broken down to smaller ones and gradually eliminated over t/2 of 17 days.

ADR: Vomiting, fever, itching, chills, swelling of salivary glands, urticaria, periorbital edema, bronchospasm, anaphylaxis.

Available as 6% Hydroxyethyl starch 100 to 500 ml.

TRADE NAME: EXPAN (6% injection).

HYOSCINE N- BUTYL BROMIDE

Indian essential medicine enlisted drug.

Scopolamine or hyoscine is rapid onset, short duration of action naturally occurring anti-cholinergic drug used for:

i. Adjunct to anesthetic.
ii. Antiemetic.
iii. Mydriatic and cycloplegic.
iv. Sedative and hypnotic.
v. Parkinsonism.

It should not be given with dextroamphetamine which may produce hallucinogenic reaction.

Hyoscine is rapidly absorbed from G.I.T. penetrates cornea.

Available as homatropine 0.3 and 0.5 mg oral, I.M. or transdermal patch.

IBUPROFEN

Enlisted both in WHO and Indian essential medicine list.

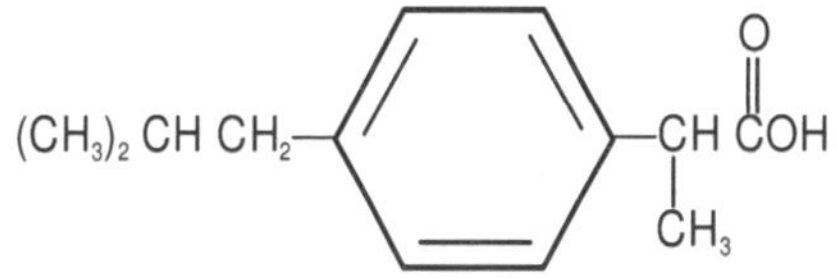

This NSAID is phenyl propionic acid derivative has analgesic anti-inflammatory action.

It is orally absorbed, peak plasma level occurs in 1-2 hours and if taken with food absorption is slowed. It is metabolized by hydroxylation and carboxylation and excreted unchanged with urine and with its metabolites. It is better tolerated.

ADR: Nausea, vomiting, diarrhoea, constipation, heart burn, epigastric pain, dizziness, light headedness, rash, amblyopia. Rise in SGPT and alkaline phosphatase, hyperuricaemia may occur.

Available as 200, 400, 600 mg tab; 100 mg/5 ml syrup.

Dose: 5-10 mg/kg.

TRADE NAME: BRUFEN, IBUGESIC, IBUSYNTH.

IMIPENEM + CILASTATIN

This is WHO enlisted combination antibiotic. Imipenem is potent and broad spectrum carbapenem antibiotic (β - lactam), spectrum includes, gram positive, cocci, Enterobacteriaceae, *Pseudomonas aeruginosa, Listeria, Bact fragilis, Cl difficile.*

The limiting features of this antibiotic is its rapid hydrolysis by enzyme dihydropeptidase I located in brush border of renal tubular cells, so if combined with cilastatin which is a reversable inhibtitor of dihydropeptidase I both have matched pharmacokinetics (t/2/hour) to protect this hydrolysis.

Dose: 0.5 g I.V. QDS (upto 4 gm/day).

Used for hospital acquired infections, infections in neutropenic, cancer and AIDS patient.

IMIPRAMINE

Enlisted in Indian essential medicine list.

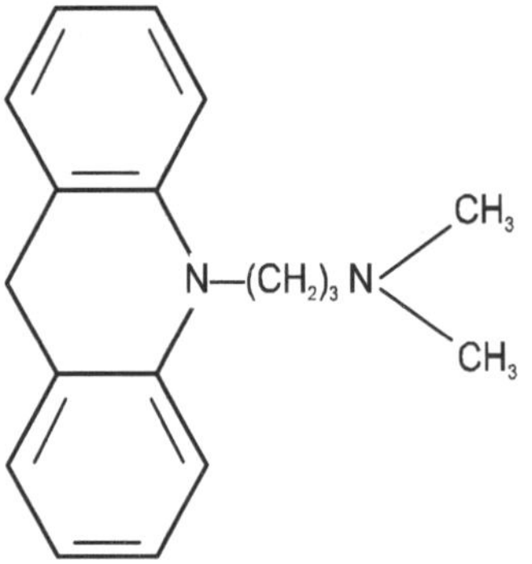

It is a prototype of tricyclic compounds more effective in treating endogenous than reactive type of defects. It inhibits norepinephrine transporter and serotonin transporter at neuronal and platelet membrane.

It is orally absorbed, bound to plasma and tissue proteins Inactivated by methylation some active metabolite like desipramine also occurs and inactivated by oxidation and glucuronide conjugation which is excreted with urine. It shows therapeutic window phenomenon (Plasma concentration 50-200 ng/ml) above and below which its effects are sub optimal.

Dose: 50-200 mg/day.

Available as 25 mg tab and 75 mg SR cap; 12.5 mg/ml in 2 ml injection.

ADR: CVS: Orthostatic hypotension, palpitation, tachycardia, arrhythmia. **CNS** confusion, Parkinsonism, delusion, hallucination, nightmare, paraesthesia. **Allergy:** Rash, urticaria, photosensitization, oedema, anticholinergic effects are: dry mouth, blurred vision, hyperhydrosin, constipation, paralytic ileus, urinary retention, aggravation of glaucoma.

Blood: Agranulocytosis, bone marrow depression. **G.I.T.:** Nausea, vomiting, stomatitis, peculiar taste, diarrhoea.

Endocrine: Testicular swelling, gynaecomastia, impotence, galactorrhoea and breast enlargement in female, decreased libido, hypo or hyperglycaemia.

Miscellaneous: Dizziness, fatigue, drowsiness, obstructive jaundice, withdrawl symptoms if withdrawn abruptly (as headache, malaise and anorexia).

TRADE NAME: DEPSONIL; ANTIDEP.

IMMUNOGLOBULIN (HUMAN)

WHO enlisted essential drug.

This is concentrated IgG obtained from pooled human plasma by fractionation in cold form.

Therapeutic Uses: Hepatitis A and B (prophylactic), measles, mumps, polio and chicken pox, agammaglobinaemia in premature infants, to augment the response of antibiotics in debilitated patient with bacterial infection.

Dose: 0.02 – 1 ml/kg I.M.

Available as 10%, 16.5% injection in 1-2 ml ampoules.

TRADE NAME: GAMMALIN; GLOBUNAL.

INDINAVIR

WHO and Indian essential medicine enlisted drug.

This is protease inhibitor, effective in HIV infection, given on empty stomach or with ritonavir, 60% bioavailable, penetrates CSF and excreted with feces.

ADR: Nephrolithiasis, jaundice (Adequate water should be taken), thrombocytopenia, raised serum aminotransferase, nausea, diarrhoea, insulin resistance may occur. It inhibits CYP3A4.

Dose: 800 mg TDS (BD if taken with 100 mg RTV).

Available as 400 mg caps.

TRADE NAME: INDIVAN; INDIVIR; VIRODIN.

INFLUENZA VACCINE

WHO enlisted essential medicine.

This viral vaccine contains inactivated virus or viral components. Give I.M. immunization may be done annually or during epidemics with 2 injections 0.5 – 1 ml in 2 months apart. Since influenza virus undergoes frequent antigenic changes its role or efficacy as vaccine is inconsistent.

Indications for inactivated virus vaccines are:

i. Adults > 50 years.
ii. High risk persons viz. asthma.
iii. Heath care workers, residents of nursing home.

iv. Children aged 6-23 months.

Live attenuated influenza virus is also available which is given to healthy person desiring protection (5-49 years). It is given intranasally.

ADR of inactivated virus vaccine: Local tenderness, fever, malaise, myalgia, allergic reaction to egg proteins.

INSULIN INJECTION (SOLUBLE)

It is included in WHO and Indian essential medicine list.

It is buffered solution of unmodified insulin stabilized by small amount of zinc. Given subcutaneous when insulin monomers are released. Peak action occurs after 2-4 hours. It is not suitable for constant basal level of sugar control so a long acting retard preparation is given simultaneously.

INTERMEDIATE ACTING (LENTE/NPH) INSULIN

LENTE is large particle, intermediate acting.

In NPH (Neutral protamine hagedorn) a protamine is added in a quantity just sufficient to complex all insulin molecules, pH is neutral, appearance cloudy, peak action at 8-10 hours on subcutaneous injection, the complex dissociates slowly.

Available as:

i. Soluble insulin 40 IU/ml; 100 IU/ml for I.V. or subcutaneous.
ii. Lente insulin (7:3) 40 IU/ml subcutaneous.
iii. Isophane (NPH) insulin 40 IU/ml for subcutaneous.

ADR of insulin: Hypoglycaemia, local reaction, allergy, edema.

Therapeutic Uses:

i. Diabetes mellitus (not controlled by diet, primary and secondary failure, under weight) to tide infection, trauma, surgery, pregnancy.
ii. Ketoacidosis.
iii. Non-ketotic hyperosmolar hyperglycaemic coma.

INTRAPERITONEAL DIALYSIS SOLUTION

Included both in WHO and Indian essential medicine list.

Peritoneal dialysis is widely available easily instituted method using hard PVC catheter into peritoneal space using trochar through scalpel skin stab. It may continuous ambulatory peritoneal dialysis (CAPD). Three to five exchanges required per day.

Indication:

i. Uraemia severe.
ii. CRF for support untill long term dialysis is started.

Complication: Pain, leakage, infection.

Composition: Na^+ 135 mmol L^{-1}; Cl^- 105 mmol L^{-1}; K = 0 mmol L^{-1}, glucose 80 mmol L^{-1}, Ca^{2+} 1.75 mmol/L^{-1}, Mg 0.50 mmol L^{-1}; lactate 35 $mmol^{-1}$.

Higher concentration of glucose is used if fluid needs to be removed.

IODINE

WHO and Indian essential medicine enlisted drug.

Iodine is an element which is a constituents of thyroid hormone, is fatest acting thyroid inhibitors.

It is therapeutically used for:

i. Deficiency states.
ii. In hyperthyroidism.
iii. As antiseptic.
iv. As expectorant.
v. Dermatological agents.
vi. In contrast media.

Acute iodine intoxication (either for suicide or accidental intake) produces iodism manifested as organ that incorporate iodine (viz. thyroid, salivary glands, eye) and other symptoms are edema, fever, conjunctivitis, lymphadenopathy, laryngeal edema.

Preparations available are:

i. Lugol's solution 5% iodine in potassium iodide solution.
ii. Colloidal iodine 10% (5-10 drops/day).
iii. Colossal 8 mg iodine/5 ml.

Radio-active iodine is used for hyperthyroidism of Graves' disease and toxic nodular goitre.

IPRATROPIUM BROMIDE

WHO enlisted essential medicine.

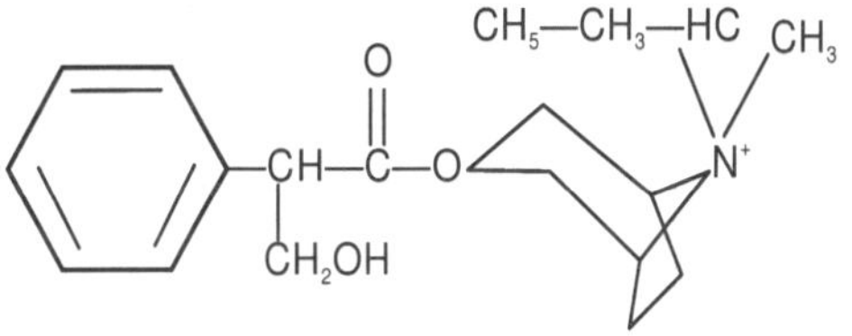

It is quaternary amines used for asthma (semisynthetic derivative).

Given as 40-80 μg by inhalation puff, which acts selectively on bronchial muscles, without altering volume and constituents of respiratory tract and without any depressant clearance by bronchial epithelium. It is more suitable for regular prophylactic which lasts for 4-6 hours. More effective of COPD than bronchial asthma.

ADR: Dry mouth, cough, bad taste, systemic side effects are less because of poor absorption.

Doses: 20 μg – 40 μg / puff, 2 puffs TDS to QDS; 250 μg/ml respiratory solution 0.4 to 2 ml nebulised solution with β_2 agonist.

0.084% nasal spray for perennial rhinitis.

Available as IPRAVENT (Inhaler, respiratory solution) or IPRANASE AQ 0.084% nasal spray.

IRON DEXTRAN

This is enlisted both in WHO and Indian essential medicine list.

It is colloidal solution containing 50 mg of elemental iron/ml indicated in:

i. Patient cannot tolerate G.I. iron.
ii. Failure to absorb iron (malabsorption).
iii. Non-compliance.
iv. Severe deficiency with chronic bleeding.
v. Along with erythropoietin because oral iron may not be absorbed at sufficient rate to fulfil the demand of erythropoisis.

Other information is mentioned with ferrous salts.

ISOFLURANE

Enlisted in Indian essential medicine list.

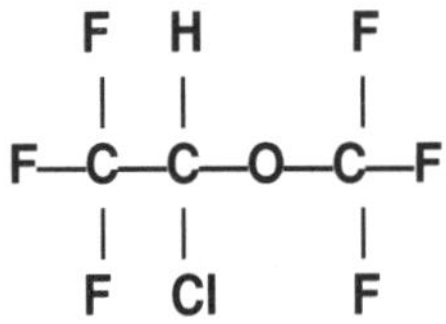

It is an isomer of enflurane a substitute of halothane, but more potent, more volatile and less soluble in blood. Induction and recovery is rapid. 1.5-3% induces anaesthesia given by special vaporizer in 7-10 minutes, 1-2% is used for maintenance.

ADR: BP may fall, tachycardia, respiratory depression (assistant required), secretions are increased. It does not provoke seizure, routinely used but costly.

TRADE NAME: SOFANE.

ISONIAZID

WHO and Indian essential medicine enlisted drug.

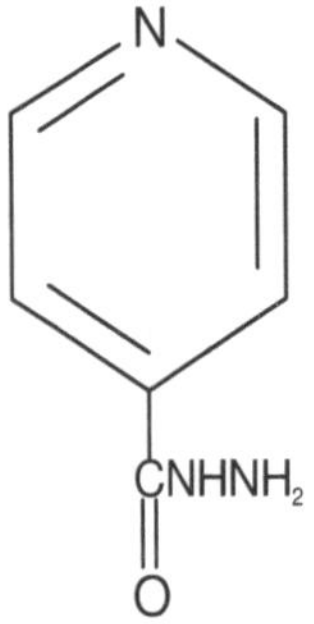

Perhaps this synthetic compound is best anti-tubercular first line drug in respect to therapeutic efficacy, toxicity, cost, patient acceptance and ease of administration. It is used in combination with other anti-tubercular agents has resulted in pronounced changes in all aspects of the disease.

Dose: 4-5 mg/kg once daily orally generally, may be given perenterally in same dose if oral dose is not practical. In Tb meningitis or disseminated Tb or in rapid acetylator it may be given in the dose of 10-20 mg/kg/day.

It is completely absorbed orally, penetrates all tissues and tubercular cavities, placenta, meninges, metabolized in liver by acetylation and excreted with urine. Some are slow and some are fast acetylators.

ADR:

- Peripheral meningitis (paraesthesia, numbness, convulsion, mental disturbances due to pyridoxine B_6 utilization) so B_6 should be given simultaneously prophylactically).
- Hepatitis.
- Rash.
- Fever.
- Acne.
- Arthralgia.

Interactions: Phenytoin, carbamazepine, diazepam and warfarin's metabolism is inhibited by it.

Its combinations pack:

i. Ethambutol.
ii. Rifampicin.
iii. Rifampicin and pyrazinamide.
iv. Rifampicin, pyrazinamide and ethambutol are enlisted with WHO enlisted essential drugs which are discussed as individual drug.

ISOPRENALINE

Enlisted in Indian essential medicine list.

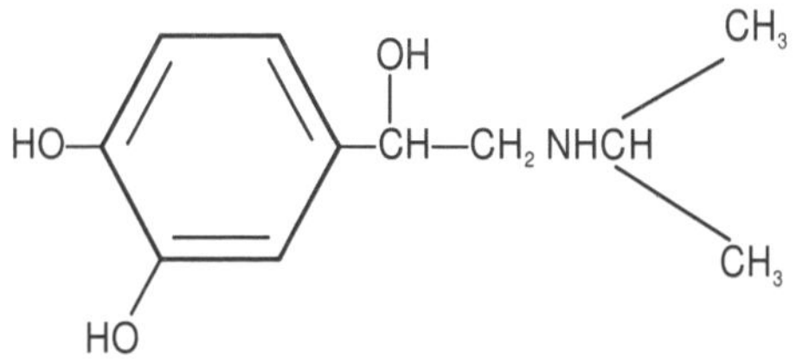

Isoprenaline is catecholamine which relieves broncho-constriction, other effects are relaxation of G.I. smooth muscle, increasing rate and force of cardiac contraction. Inhalation preparation is preferred for asthmatics but it can also be given sublingually.

ADR: Palpitation, tachycardia, hypotension, tremor, nervousness, precipitation of angina, excessive inhalation may cause refractory bronchial obstruction and sudden death, tolerance, refractoriness.

Therapeutic Uses:

i. To maintain idioventricular rate till pacemaker is implanted.

ii. Bronchial asthma.

Dose: 20 mg S/L; 1-2 mg I.M.; 5-10 microgram/min I.V. infusion.

For oral inhalation careful instruction of the patient for proper use of the device preferably by demonstration is essential. If nebulizer is used. With any nebulized preparation, the least number of inhalation of the most diluted solution necessary to obtain relief is desirable and children should use the nebulizer in presence of knowledgable adults. For nebulizer breath should be withheld in full inhalation following complete exhalation.

Dose: 5 to 15 deep inhalation of a mist of 1: 200 solutions. When oxygen aerosol preparation upto 0.5 ml of 1: 200 solution is given with an oxygen flow of 4 liters for 15 – 20 minutes. For powdered inhalation 2-4 inhalation of normal force and depth is allowed.

TRADE NAMES: ISOPRIN 4 mg/2 ml inj; NEOEPININE 20 mg S/L tabs.

ISOSORBIDE DINITRATE

Enlisted in WHO essential medicine list.

This drug is solid. It can be used similar to nitroglycerine sublingually at the time of attack. Slightly slower in action. It is orally absorbed as well for chronic prophylaxis but presystemic metabolism on oral administration is pronounced and variable but with sustained release preparation this effect is protected (6-10 hours protection). The last dose should not be taken after 6 pm to allow nitrate level to fall during sleep at night.

Available as 5,10 mg tab; 20 and 40 mg S.R. tab.

TRADE NAME: SORBITRATE; DITRATE SR tab.

ISOSORBIDE 5 MONONITRATE

Enlisted in Indian essential medicine list.

This agent available as tablet form, does not undergo significant first pass metabolism therefore its oral bio-availablity is excellent. Its t/2 is longer than isosorbide dinitrate and it is available as plain and sustained release tab. Last dose is taken in the afternoon and SR tab once in the morning.

TRADE NAME: MONOTRATE 10, 20, 40 mg tab; 25 and 50 mg SR tabs.

ISOXSUPRINE

Indian essential medicine enlisted drug.

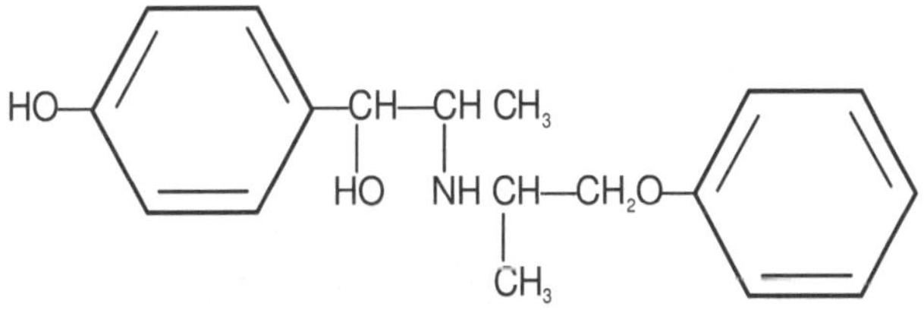

Though it is classified as beta adrenoreceptor stimulant but in animal studies it indicates that its vascular effects are direct action. It increases muscular blood flow in patient of occlusive vascular diseases to relieve intermittent claudication.

Therapeutic Uses:

i. Intermittent claudication and vasospastic diseases.
ii. Cerebrovascular disease.
iii. Dysmenorrhea.
iv. Threatened abortion.
v. Premature labour.

Available as 10, 20 mg tab; 5 mg/ml in 2 ml container.

Dose: 10-20 mg TDS to QDS.

Intramuscular 5 to 10 mg BD to QDS.

ADR: Dizziness, Hypotension, Tachycardia, Rash.

TRADE NAME: DUVADILAN.

ISPHAGULA

Enlisted in Indian essential medicine list.

It is natural colloidal mucilage which after absorption of water forms gelatinous mass and acts as bulk purgative. Don't ask the patient to swallow dry because it may cause esophageal impaction. It acts on 1-3 days.

Dose: 3-12 gram.

Available as isphagula husk refined 27 g/30 g.

TRADE NAME: NATURE CARE.

IUD CONTAINING COPPER

WHO and Indian essential medicine enlisted drug.

Intrauterine devices (IUD) can be divided into:

i. Medicated; and
ii. Unmedicated IUD. Copper IUD are medicated IUD belongs to 2nd generation IUD (First generation are unmedicated and 3rd generation are hormone containing).

The earlier devices of copper T IUD were copper 7; Copper T 200; Newer devices are variants of the T device:

i. T Cu – 220 C.
ii. T Cu – 380 A or Ag.
iii. Nova T.
iv. Multiload devices of (a) ML Cu 250 (b) ML Cu 375.

The newer copper are more effective. The number included in the devices refer to surface area in sq inches. Nova T and T- Cu 380 Ag contains silver core upon which copper wire is wrapped.

Advantages:

i. Expulsion rate is low.
ii. Pain and bleeding is less.
iii. Easy to fit even in nullipara.
iv. More effective even as post coital contraceptives.

IVERMECTIN

WHO enlisted essential medicine.

This semisynthetic antinematode principle is obtained from *Streptomyces avermitilis*. It is drug of choice. Its uses are:

i. Onchocerciasis (single dose).
ii. Strongyloidosis.
iii. Bancroftian and Brugian filaria.
iv. Cutaneous larva migrans.
v. Moderately sensitive to enterobius.
vi. Trichuris.
vii. It kills head lice; and
viii. Scabies.

It produces tonic paralysis to nematodes through special types of glutamate gated Cl^- channel present in invertebrates.

Orally absorbed, widely distributed but does not penetrate CNS, sequestered in liver and fat with long t/2 of 48 to 60 hours.

ADR: Pruritis, Giddiness, Nausea, Abdominal pain, Constipation, Lethargy, E.C.G. changes, Reaction due to degeneration products of microfilaria.

Dose: 10-15 mg single (0.2 mg/kg) orally. It has replaced diethyl carbamazine citrate for onchocerciasis and is included in river blindness control programme.

Available as 3 and 6 mg tabs.

TRADE NAME: IVERMECTOL.

KANAMYCIN

It is an aminoglycoside antibiotic obtained from *S.Kanamyceticus.* It is more toxic to cochlea and kidney. Hearing loss is more common. Occasionally used as 2nd line drug in drug resistance tuberculosis.

Dose: 0.5 g I.M., BD to TDS.

KETAMINE

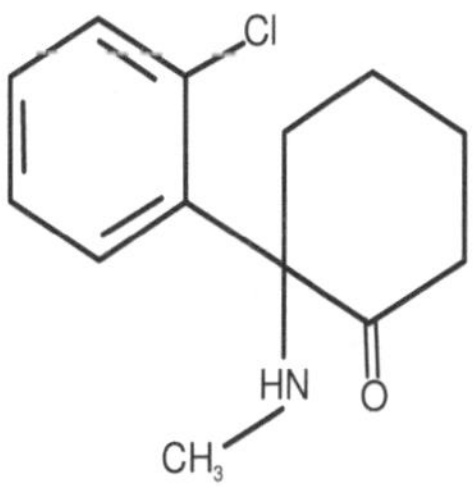

It is a recemic mixture of S (+) and R (-) optical isomer pharmacologically related to phencyclidine produces dissociative anesthetic state characterized by catatonia, amnesia, analgesia with or without loss of consciousness.

It blocks excitatory neurotransmitter glutamic acid at NMDA receptor. Primarily in cortex and sub cortex. It does not depress respiration. It causes dose related cardiovascular stimulation. It increases cerebral blood flow, oxygen consumption and intracranial pressure. Respiration is not depressed, airway reflexes are maintained, muscle tone increases.

Available as 50 mg/ml in 2 ml amp. Dose 1-3 mg/kg. Recovery starts after 10-15 minutes. Patient remains amnesic for 1-2 hours. It is metabolized in liver children tolerate it better.

It is used for poor risk geriatric patient and high risk cardiogenic and septic patient because of cardiostimulatory properties. In children it is used with propofol for painful procedures. S (+) ketamine is more anesthetic and analgesic.

KETOCONAZOLE

It is included in essential medicine list 2003 of India.

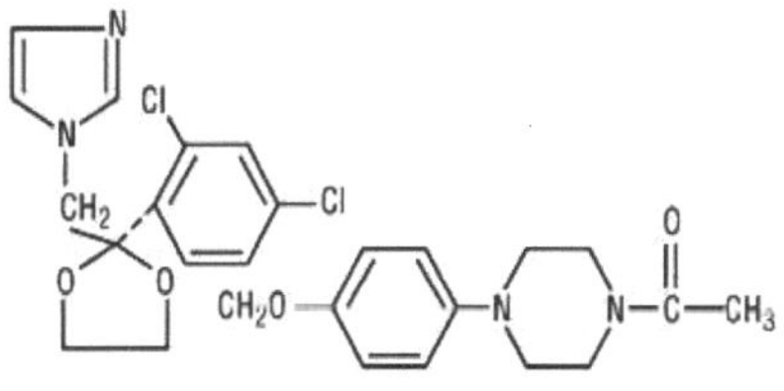

It belongs to imidazole group of antifungal drug used orally. It is also found to kill leishmania by inhibiting conversion of lanosterol to ergosterol and its membrane function is impaired. It is used as add on drug for kala azar in the dose of 600 mg O.D. for 4 weeks. Antifungal dose is 200 mg OD to BID. Its penetration to CSF is poor.

Nausea, vomiting, loss of appetite, headache, rash, decreases androgen production in testes. It inhibits CYP3A4 and raises blood level of Phenytin, Digoxin, Diazepam, Warfarin, Statin. Polymorphic and ventricular tachycardia can occur with cisapride, terfenadine and astemizole. Since it inhibits mammalian cytochrome P450 more than fungal P450, it is withdrawn from USA market.

It is also used to treat Cushing's syndrome to decrease corticosteroid production.

It may be used topically as cream. 2% shampoo is used for dandruff.

LAMIVUDINE (3TC)

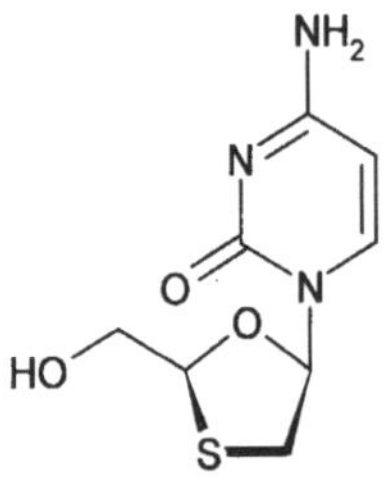

This nucleoside reverse transcriptase inhibitor is anti-retroviral agent. It is a cytosine analog with synergistic activity with different anti-retroviral nucleoside analogs. It is phosphorylated intracellularly and inhibits reverse transcriptase of HIV and HBV. Systemic toxicity is low. Resistance occurs due to mutation, cross resistance with didanosine is noted with HIV.

Orally absorbed, food does not interfere absorption, excreted unchanged with urine.

ADR: Headache, Fatigue, Nausea, Anorexia, Abdominal pain, Pancreatitis, Neuropathy.

Dose:

i. Chronic hepatitis B 100 mg OD.
ii. HIV infection 150 mg BD.

Available as: 100, 150 mg tab, 150 mg/5 ml solution.
TRADE NAME: LAMIVIR; HEPTAVIR.

LAMIVUDINE + ZIDOVUDINE

This drug combination is enlisted in both WHO and Indian essential medicine list.

LAMIVUDINE + NEVIRAPINE + STAVUDINE

This triple drug combination is enlisted in both WHO and Indian essential medicine list.

L-ASPARAGINASE

Enlisted both in WHO and Indian essential medicine list.

Asparaginase (L-asparagine amidohydrolase) is an enzyme to treat childhood acute lymphocytic leukemia. This drug is isolated from and purified from bacterial culture. The enzyme L-asparaginase degrades to L-asparagine to L-aspartic acid and deprives the leukemic cells an essential metabolite and cause their death. The remission produced by it for leukemia is short lasting.

ADR: Anaphylaxis, liver damage, pancreatitis.

Dose: 50-200 KU/kg I.V. daily × 2-4 weeks.

Available as 10000 KU/vial.

TRADE NAME: LEUNASE.

LEVAMISOLE

Enlisted in WHO's essential medicine list.

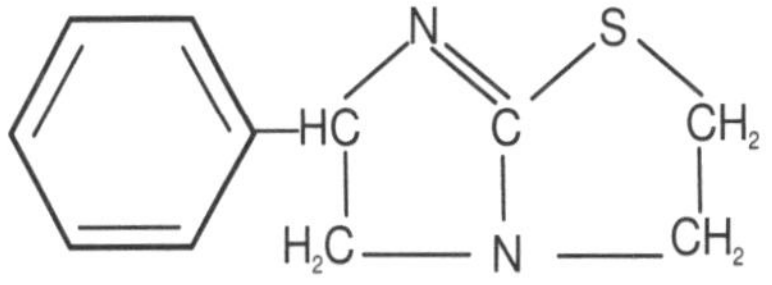

Levamisole is levo isomer of tetramisole. It is white, crystalline, water soluble hydrochloride of 2,3,5,6 tetrahydro 6 phenyl imidazo (2,1b) thiazole.

Therapeutic Uses: Ascarasis and Ancylostomiasis, Strongyloides larvae are killed.

It causes tonic paralysis and expulsion of live worms and interferes with carbohydrate metabolism.

Dose for Ascaris: 50 mg for children (10-19 kg).
100 mg for children 20-39 kg.
150 mg for over 40 kgs.

It is second choice for *A duodenale:* Two doses at 12 hours.

Available as 50 and 150 mg tab; 50 mg/5 ml syrup.

ADR: Nausea, Abdominal pain, Fatigue, Giddiness Drowsiness and Insomnia.

Other important effect of levamisole are immunomodulation because it restores the depressed T cell function, used as disease

modifying agent in Rheumatoid arthritis, in malignancies, Aphthous ulcers. Repeated doses produce severe reactions.
TRADE NAME: VERMISOL; DEWORMIS.

LEVODOPA AND CARBIDOPA

This combination preparation is enlisted in WHO and Indian essential medicine list.

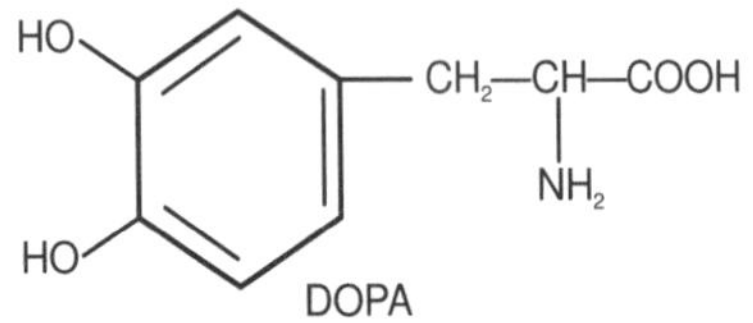

DOPA

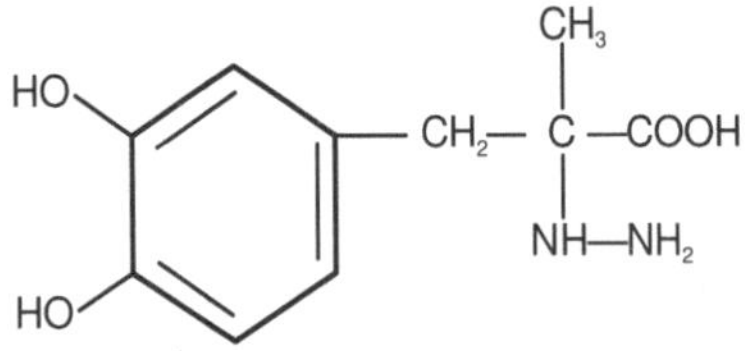

Dopamine cannot cross the BBB so does not have therapeutic value. Dihydroxy phenyl alanine can enter BBB via L-amino acid transporter (LAT) and decarboxylated to dopamine to be effective in Parkinsonism.

Carbidopa is peripheral decarboxylase inhibitors, increases dopamine concentration in the brain and this combination preparation.

i. Prolong t/2 of levodopa, decreases systemic level of dopamine and minimizes its cardiac complications.
ii. Degree of improvement is more with less "on off" phenomenon.

It is orally absorbed with high first pass metabolism, t/2 1-2 hours decarboxylated and the metabolites are excreted with urine.

ADR of Levodopa: Nausea, Vomiting, Postural hypotension, Exacerbation of angina, Altered taste sensation, Cardiac arrhythmia, Abnormal movements (Tics, tongue thrusting, grimacing, behavioral effects (Anxiety, nightmare); "on off" phenomenon. Should be given with caution in IHD; cerebrovascular patients, peptic ulcer, glaucoma, hepatic and kidney diseases.

Available as 0.5 g tab.

Dose: 0.25 BD after meals.

Sinemet is combination product of levodopa and carbidopa in the ratio of 10.1 Apart from reducing the dose of levodopa it decreases incidence of nausea, vomiting the dyskinetic and psychiatric disturbances appear early and may be more with Sinemet.

Available as	Trade name
Levodopa + Carbidopa 100 mg + 70 mg	Sinemet, Duodopa 110 Syndopa

Dose: 1 tab BD to QDS.

Like all fixed dose combinations, Sinemet may not be suitable for all patients.

TRADE NAME OF LEVODOPA: LEVOPA.

LEVONORGESTREL

Enlisted in WHO essential medicine list.

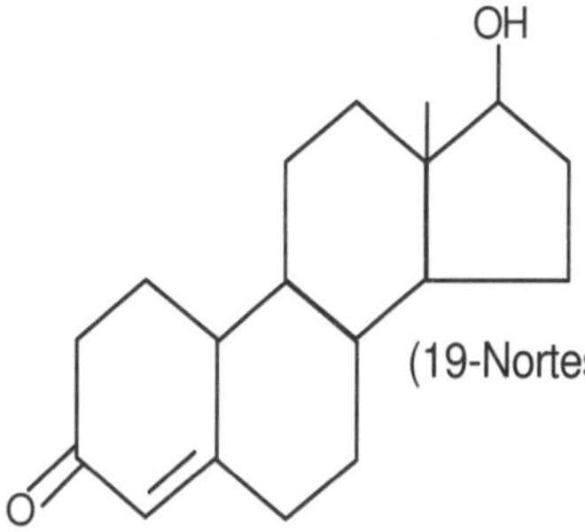

(19-Nortestosterone derivative)

This is a synthetic progestin, chemically 19-Nortestosterone derivative. The progesterone preparations are used for:

i. Contraceptives.
ii. Hormone replacement therapy.
iii. DUB.
iv. Endometriosis.
v. Post menopausal syndrome/Tension.
vi. Threatened or habitual abortion.
vii. Endometrial ca (high doses).

ADR: 19-Nortestosterone derivative can cause nausea, breast discomforts, headache, fatigue, mental depression, liver damage apart from their pharmacological actions which modify the menstrual cycle.

Contraindications are: Uterine and breast cancer, thrombo-embolic disorder, undiagnosed vaginal bleeding, porphyria, pregnancy, hepatic disorder.

Available as 0.75 mg tab.

In Norplant 6 capsules with 36 mg levonorgestrel (Total 216 mg) is implanted subcutaneously which protects pregnancy for 5 years.

TRADE NAME: NORLEVO.

LEVOTHYROXINE

WHO and Indian essential medicine enlisted drug.

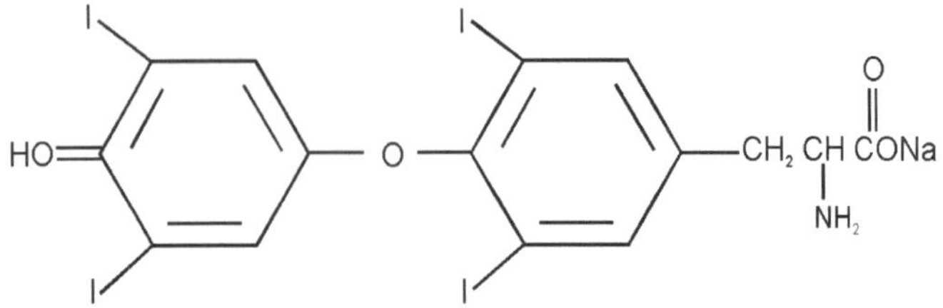

This is synthetic sodium salt of levorotatory isomer of tetraiodothyronine (thyroxine).

It is orally absorbed, bioavailability is 75% but decreased in severe hypothyroidism. Should be given on empty stomach. Its metabolism is enhanced by enzyme inducer. Its onset of action slower. In myexedema coma should be given I.V.

ADR: Of overdose viz. tachycardia, palpitation, raised pulse pressure, angina pectoris, tremor, nervousness, insomnia, leg cramps, headache, change of apetite,vomiting, diarrhea, intolerance to heat, hyperhydrosis.

Therapeutic Uses: Replacement therapy; goitre, myxedema coma, chronic lymphocytic thyroidits. To obviate goitrogenic effect (of lithium carbonate, PAS, sulfonamide). Thyroid nodule, papillary carcinoma of thyroid.

Empirical Uses: Refractory anaemia, chronic non healing ulcer, menstrual disorder, obstinate constipation.

Available as 25; 50; 100 microgram tabs.

Dose: 0.05 to 0.1 mg daily to increase every 2-3 weeks until desired effect is observed. In older patient start with 0.0125 to 0.25 mg and then increase after 6-8 weeks till response is achieved. In children dose should not increase 0.05 mg. Injection preparation are also available.

TRADE NAME: ELTROXIN; THYRONORM; ROXIN.

LIDOCAINE (LIGNOCAINE)

WHO and Indian essential medicine enlisted drug.

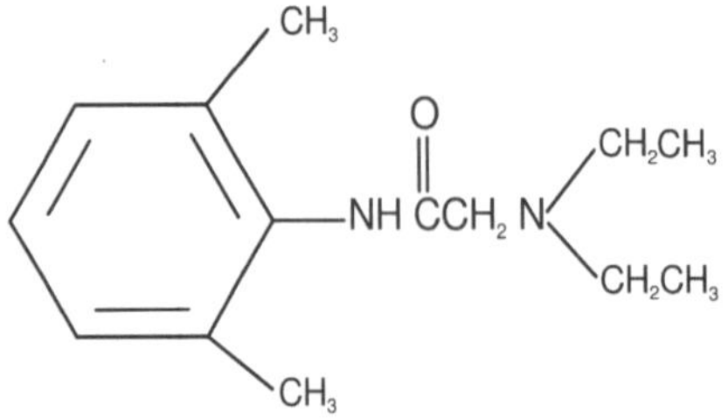

This is amide linked local anesthetic (both surface and injections) available in variety of forms. It blocks nerve conduction within 3 minutes when injected around it. It has also class IB anti-arrhythmic effect.

It is inactive orally, has to be given I.V. because of first pass metabolism. It is hydrolysed deethylated and conjugated and the metabolites are excreted with urine. Its metabolism is hepatic blood flow dependent.

ADR: Drowsiness, nausea, paresthesia, blurred vision, nystagmus, twitching, B.P. may fall, coma, respiratory arrest.

Therapeutic Uses: Ventricular tachyarrhythmia (in emergencies like MI, cardiac surgery), digitalis toxicity.

ANTI-ARRHYTHMIC LIGNOCAINE

Dose: 50-100 mg I.V. bolus followed by 20-40 mg every 20 min or 1-3 mg/minutes.

Available as 20 mg/ml in 5-50 ml vial.

TRADE NAME: XYLOCARD; GESICARD.

LOCAL ANAESTHETIC LIGNOCAINE

4% topical solution; 2% jelly; 5% oint, 1% and 2% injections with or without adrenaline, 5% heavy for spinal anaesthesia, as nasal spray 1-4%.

TRADE NAME: XYLOCAINE; GESICAIN.

LIDOCAINE WITH EPINEPHRINE

This combination is also enlisted both in WHO and Indian essential medicine list.

Generally with 1:50000 to 1:200000 in 50 ml multi dose container or 30 ml single dose container. Aqueous solutions without epinephrine can be autoclaved repeatedly. Solutions with dextrose should not be autoclaved more than twice. All preparations with epinephrine contain sodium metabisulfite and all multiple dose container contain methylparaben 1mg.

LITHIUM CARBONATE

The antimaniac (mood stabilizer) lithium is small monovalent cation, effects Na, Ca, Mg metabolism and inhibits action of ADH and alters catecholamine metabolism.

It is absorbed orally slowly, not metabolized first, distributed extracellularly then gradually enters cell and penetrates brain. Its apparent vol. of distribution is 0.8L/kg. It is handled by kidney like Na.

ADR: Nausea, vomiting, diarrhea, thirst, polyuria, fine tremor, giddiness, ataxia, motor incoordination, nystagmus, mental confusion, slurred speech, hyperreflexia, goitre, diabetes insipidus. Treatment of Lithium toxicity: Symptomatic, osmotic diuretic, $NaHCO_3$; haemodialysis if level are more than 4 m Eq/L.

Contraindication: Pregnancy, sick sinus syndrome.

Therapeutic Uses: Acute mania, prophylaxis to bipolar disorder, unipolar depression, cluster headache, major depression and cancer chemotherapy induced leukopenia, inappropriate ADH secretion syndrome.

Available as 300 mg tabs, 400 mg SR tab.

Dose: 600 mg/day gradually increased to get therapeutic yield which is mostly 1200 mg/day.

TRADE NAME: LICAB; LITHOSUN.

LOCAL ANAESTHETIC/ASTRINGENT ANTI-INFLAMMATORY (ANTIHAEMORRHOIDAL)

Lidocaine 3%, hydrocortisone acetate 0.25% zinc oxide 5%, allantoin 0.5% all w/w used for haemorrhoids, anal fissure, proctitis and periproctitis.

To be applied thrice daily.

This preparation goes near to the said composition.

LOPERAMIDE

This drug is enlisted in Indian essential medicine list.

Loperamide is piperidine butyramide derivative with activity on μ receptor acts as anti-diarrhoeal. It penetrates CNS poorly and slows the G.I. motility by affecting circular and longitudinal muscles of intestine. Little tolerance develops. It also increases anal sphincters tone. It has anti-secretory effect against cholera toxins and some forms of E. coli toxins. It is OTC product. Its action starts quickly after oral dose, metabolized in liver.

Dose: 4 mg initially followed by 2 mg after each purge upto 16 mg initially followed by 2 mg after each purge upto 16 mg if clinical improvement does not occur within 48 hours, it should be stopped, it should not to be prescribed below 2 years.

Dose: Upto 3 mg for 2-5 years of age.
Upto 4 mg for 6-8 years of age.
Upto 6 mg for 8-12 years of age.

TRADE NAME: IMODIUM.

LOPINAVIR

This is WHO enlisted essential medicine.

This protease inhibitor acts against anti-retrovirus which is available only in combination with ritonavir (discussed elsewhere) to improve bioavailability in ratio of lopinavir 100/ritonavir 400.

Dose: 1 BD after or with meal. These sub therapeutic doses of ritonavir inhibit the CYP3A mediated metabolism of lopinavir resulting increasing exposure of lopinavir (pharmacokinetic enchancer) and decreasing emergence of resistance and increases patients compliance.

ADR: Diarrhea, pain abdomen, nausea, vomiting, asthenia.
TRADE NAME: RITOMAX-L.

LOPINAVIR + RITONAVIR

This is a WHO enlisted essential drug combination.

LOSARTAN

Enlisted in Indian essential medicine list.

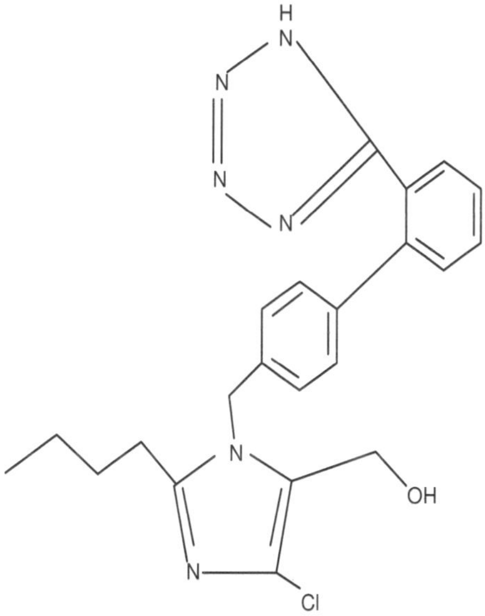

This is a competitive antagonist of angiotensin. More selective for AT_1 than AT_2 and blocks all the actions of A II (vasoconstriction) central and peripheral sympathetic stimulation, release of aldosterone and adrenaline from adrenals.

It is orally absorbed, food does not alter its absorption partly carboxylated to active metabolite, protein bound, does not enter brain and excreted with urine. Dose should be reduced in hepatic dysfunction.

ADR: Hypotension, hyperkalemia, dry cough angioedema (occasionally), headache, dizziness, fetopathic.

Dose: 50 mg OD to BD or 25 mg OD in liver diseases.

Available as 25, 50 mg tab.

Therapeutic Uses: Hypertension, CCF, myocardial infarction, diabetic nephropathy.

TRADE NAME: REPACE; GIFTAN; LOSACAR.

LUMEFANTRINE

WHO enlisted essential medicine.

This aryl alcohol is available as fixed dose combination with artemether. The t/2 of the combination is 4.5 hours. Orally absorbed, improves if taken with food.

Dose: BD. Effective in P. falciparum acting as erythrocytic schizontocides. This combination appears to have no cardiac toxicity.

ADR: Headache, dizziness, sleep distribution, abdominal pain, arthralgia, pruritis and rash. It should not be given with drug metabolized by CYP $2D_6$.

MAGNESIUM HYDROXIDE

WHO enlisted essential medicine.

It acts as an antacid. This preparation has high neutralizing capacity with rapid onset of action. Like other amphoteric antacids, the liquid preparations are more active.

Dose: Adults 300 mg to 2 gm powder or one to two tablets as often needed. Tablets should be well chewed before swallowing. Milk of magnesia 5-30 ml of liquid as needed. Children 2.5 to 5 ml.

ADR: Antacids with Mg are less likely to produce serious toxic effects except hypermagnesemia. Other side effects are diarrhoea so aluminium salts are frequently mixed with it. Ulcer patient very rarely tolerate Mg salts for a long period as sole antacids.

MAGNESIUM SULFATE

WHO and Indian essential medicine enlisted drug.

This drug has multiple actions: When given by different routes, it produces different actions.

Given by I.V. route, it is used to control convulsion and to reduce BP in a patient of toxaemia of pregnancy. It has also tocolytic action to delay preterm labour.

Dose: 2-4 gm over 10-20 minutes then 1g / hour I.V. It has also antacid property (Epsom salt) and laxative properties (osmotic purgative).

It is used per rectally to reduce intracranial tension (rarely used).

MANNITOL

Enlisted both in WHO and Indian essential medicine list.

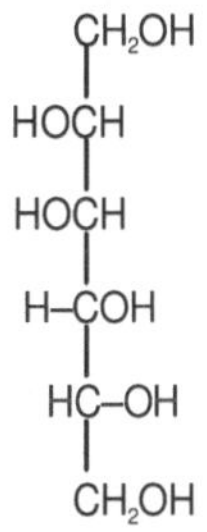

This is osmotic diuretics. It is non-electrolyte, low molecular weight (Mol wt 182) pharmacologically inert, given I.V. usually with furosemide, not metabolized in body; freely filtered at glomerulus.

It is excreted with t/2 of 0.5 to 1.5 hours.

Therapeutic Uses:

i. Raised intracranial and intraocular pressure.
ii. To maintain g.f.r in shock, trauma, cardiac surgery, hemolytic reactions.
iii. To counter osmolality of plasma and ecf due to haemolysis, peritoneal dialysis.
iv. With large volume of saline in poisoning for forced diuresis.

Contraindications: Anuria, acute tubular necrosis, pulmonary edema, CCF, left ventricular failure, cerebral haemorrhage.

ADR: Hypersensitivity, headache (due to hyponatremia, nausea, vomiting).

Available as 10% and 20% solution in 100, 350 and 500 ml bottles.

MEASLES VACCINES

Enlisted both in WHO and Indian essential medicine list.

This is life attenuated vaccine, also grown in chick embryo, available as single dose vial, which contains 1000 TCID 50 of Edmonston Schwarz strain.

TRADE NAME: ROUVAX; RIMEVAX or EDMONSTON ZAGREB; M-VAC.

Given subcutaneously over deltoid. It produces modified infection with fever, rash, coryza appears after 5-10 days. Its immunity lasts for 8 years and no booster required. Tuberculous, malnourished and chronically ill patient should be protected with it to prevent serious complications of measles. Given to epilepsy and convulsion patient cautiously.

The combinations of Measles, Mumps and Rubella vaccines are also available, given subcutaneously over deltoid in children older than 12 months.

MEBENDAZOLE

WHO and Indian essential medicine enlisted drug.

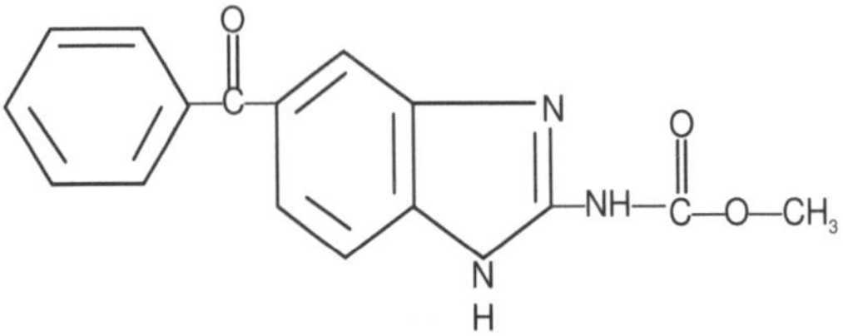

This synthetic benzimidazole has wide spectrum anti-helminth activity and fewer side effects.

Its spectrum includes round worm, pin worm, whip worm, hook worms. It is effective to a lesser extent in thread worms but it used successfully to treat Tinea infestations. Prolonged use of mebendazole regress the size of hydatid cyst.

The immobilization and lethal action of mebendazole tabs 2-3 days to develop.

It is only partly absorbed, 75-90% is passed in the faeces. The absorbed fraction is metabolized and the inactive metabolites excreted out with urine and faeces.

ADR: Abdominal pain, diarrhea, less systemic toxicity due to poor absorption. Expulsion of ascaris from mouth and nose has occurred. High doses may produce allergy, loss of hair, agranulocytosis.

Available as 100 mg chewable tabs, 100 mg/5 ml syrup.

Dose and Duration: Same above 2 years and ½ in 1-2 years of age, i.e., 1 tab BD × 3 days and for Enterobius 100 mg single dose to be repeated after 1-3 weeks. Hydatid disease 200 mg BD to TDS × 3-4 weeks. For Trichinella 200 mg BD × 4 days.

TRADE NAME: MEBEX.

MELPHALAN

Enlisted in Indian essential medicine list.

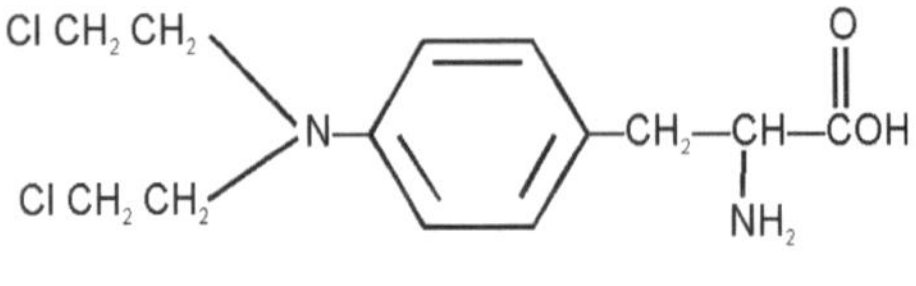

This alkylating agent, used to treat multiple myeloma, signs of improvement is evidenced by decreased in abnormal protein. Some studies show it is also effective against seminoma, Ewing sarcoma, CLL, Ovarian carcinoma, Breast carcinoma, Reticulum cell carcinoma, Polycythemia and occasionally in malignant melanoma, osteosarcoma and Burkitt's lymphoma of the jaw.

It is ineffective in acute leukemia. Its usefulness in Hodgkin's disease remains to be determined.

ADR: Bone marrow depression, aphthous ulcer, infection, diarrhoea, hemorrhage from G.I.T. pancreatitis.

Dose: 10 mg daily × 7days or 6 mg/day × 2-3 weeks a gap for a month and then 2-4 mg OD as maintenance.

Available as 2, 5 mg tab; 50 mg/vial inj.

TRADE NAME: ALKERAN.

MEDROXY PROGESTERONE ACETATE (DEPOT)

WHO enlisted essential medicine.

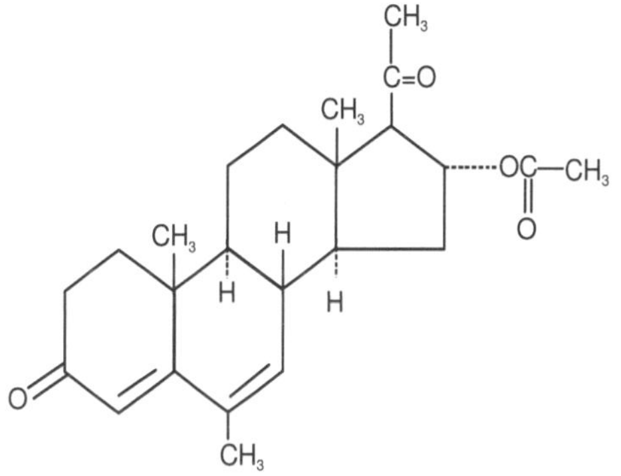

This progesterone derivative is effective orally and perenterally. Depot perenteral preparations are due to delayed systemic absorption. Priming of oestrogen is necessary for its action.

The elimination t/2 of oral preparation is 32-44 hours.

ADR: Breast engorgement, headache, swinging of mood, acne, oesophageal reflux, irregular bleeding, chances of breast cancer.

Dose: Oral 5-10 mg for secondary amenorrhea (Not due to pregnancy, DUB, dysmenorrhea, premenstrual tension).

Intramuscular: For adjunctive and palliative treatment of inoperable, recurrent metastatic endometrial carcinoma. 400 mg to 1g weekly. For endometriosis 50 mg or more weekly for 6 months; for contraception 150 mg per 6 weeks and then once in every 3 months.

Available as: 2.5, 5, 10 mg tab; 150 mg/ml injection.

TRADE NAME: FARLUTAL; PROVERA; INJ DEPOT PROVERA.

ADR: Complete disorganization of menstrual pattern, irregular bleeding.

MEDROXY PROGESTERONE ACETATE + ESTRADIOL CYPIONATE is WHO enlisted essential drug.

MEDROXY PROGESTRONE ACETATE + OESTRADIOL CYPIONATE

Enlisted in WHO's essential medicine list.

These two combinations preparations in the dose of 2.5 mg and 5 mg is used as combined hormonal injectable contraceptive given once a month. It is more than 99% effective if given in schedule and gives women a reliable and convenient new birth control option.

MEFLOQUINE

WHO enlisted essential medicine.

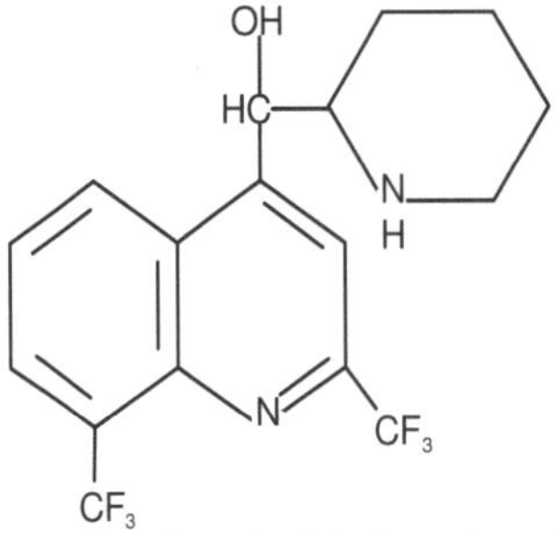

This anti-malarial drug is quinoline-methanol derivative, has developed to deal with the problem of chloroquine resistant P.falciparum. It is fast acting erythrocyte schizontocide.

It is orally slowly absorbed, plasma protein bound, concentrated in liver and lung metabolized in liver and secreted with bile t/2 2-3 weeks due to tissue binding and enterohepatic circulation.

ADR: Bitter taste, nausea, vomiting, pain abdomen, dizziness, bradycardia, disturbed balance, ataxia, errors in operating machine, strange dreams, convulsions, anxiety, rarely haematological, hepatic and cutaneous toxicities may occur. Safe after 1st trimester of pregnancy. It prolongs QTC and may cause cardiac arrest if given with halofantrine or quinidine.

Therapeutic Uses:

i. Multidrug resistant, P. falciparum.

ii. For travellers visiting multidrug resistant, P. falciparum as prophylactic.

Dose: 250 mg with excess of water.

Available as: 250 mg tab.
TRADE NAME: MEFLOTAS; FACITAL.

MEGLUMINE ANTIMONATE

WHO enlisted essential medicine.

Used to treat leismaniasis and fascioliasis given intramuscularly. It is sold as glucantime in France. It is pentavalent antimonial compound.

MELARSOPROL

It is WHO enlisted essential medicine.

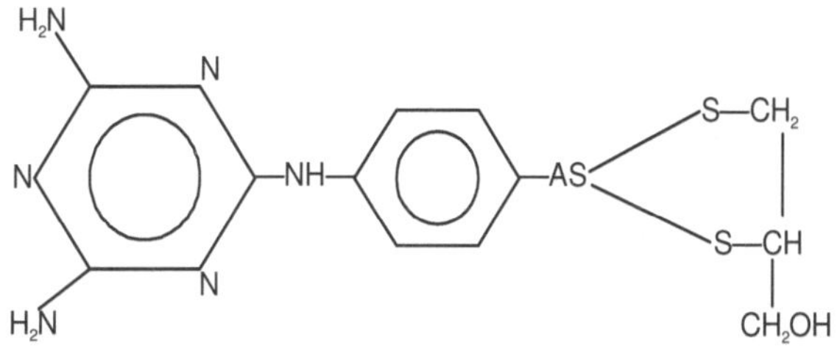

This prodrug should be given in hospital setup based on clinical assessment not on body weight in late meningoencephalitic stage of least African trypanosomiasis.

Dose: 2-3.6 mg/kg for 3-4 days with 7 days interval or continuous 10 days course of 2.2 mg/kg/day.

ADR: Fever, reactive encephalopathy, co-administration of steroids reduces incidence, hepatic and renal insufficiency, vomiting, colic's of abdomen, proteinuria, peripheral neuropathy.

MENADIONE SODIUM SULPHITE

Enlisted in Indian essential medicine.

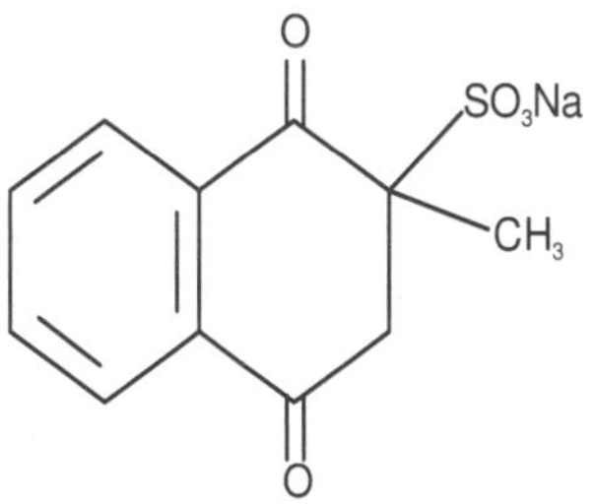

It is freely soluble in water and bile salts are not necessary for its absorption used for same purposes of vitamin K.

Available as 2.5 and 10 mg/ml in 1ml container.

Dose: Subcutaneous, I.V. or I.M. 2.5 to 10 mg daily.

MENINGOCOCCAL VACCINE

Enlisted in WHO's essential medicine list.

This vaccine contains purified capsular polysaccharide of N. meningitis group A and C 50 µg each per unit dose in 10 dose vial.

Dose: 0.5 ml S/C, I.M.

Therapeutic Uses: Prophylactically during epidemics of group A or C meningococci infection.

TRADE NAME: MENCEVAX A and C; MENINGOCOCCAL A and C.

MERCAPTOPURINE

Enlisted both in WHO and Indian essential medicine list.

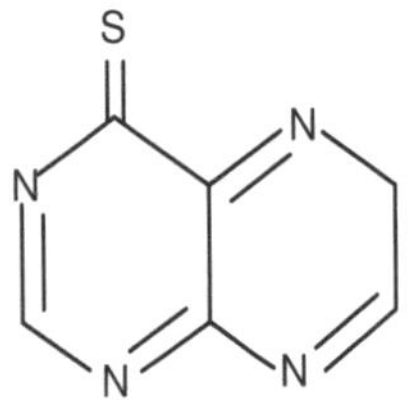

This purine antagonist anticancer drug produces complete remission in 30% of children with ALL or stem cell leukemia, when administered with prednisolone. Remission is prolonged and complete remission approaches 80%. It is also effective for choriocarcinoma and in some solid tumors.

ADR: Leucopenia, thrombocytopenia, haemorrhage, nausea, vomiting, aphthous, stomatitis, jaundice. Its dose should be reduced if given with allopurinol.

Dose: 2.5 mg/kg/day and ½ the dose for maintenance.

METFORMIN

Enlisted both in WHO and Indian essential medicine list.

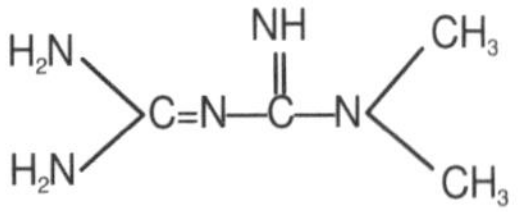

It is biguanide derivative, oral hypoglycemic agent, inhibits:

i. Hepatic gluconeogenesis.
ii. Enhances insulin mediated glucose disposal in muscle and fat cells.
iii. Inhibit absorption of glucose, hexoses, amino acids and vit B_{12} from intestine.
iv. Promote peripheral glucose utilization.
v. Reduces plasma glucagon level.

Orally absorbed, not protein bound, not metabolized and is excreted by kidney. It accumulates in renal insufficiency.

Therapeutic Uses: Type II diabetes mellitus and improves lipid profile in this condition.

ADR: Abdominal pain, anorexia, nausea, metallic taste, diarrhoea, lactic acidosis, Vit B_{12} deficiency.

Available as 0.5 and 0.85 gm tab.

Dose: 500 to 2.55 gm daily.

TRADE NAME: GLYCIPHAGE; GLYCOMET.

METHOTREXATE

WHO and Indian essential medicine enlisted drug.

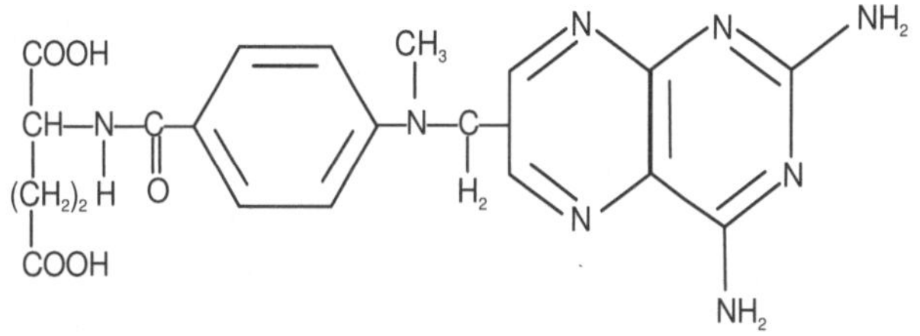

Methotrexate is an antimetabolite, inhibits dihydrofolate, reductase and thereby blocks conversion of dihydrofolic acid to tetrahydrofolic acid. It is cell cycle specific of S phase and inhibits DNA synthesis and also effects RNA and protein synthesis.

It is orally absorbed, 50% protein bound. Its toxicity increases with concurrent use of aspirin and sulfonamide both of which decreases its renal tubular secretion.

Effective for: Choriocarcinoma, chorioadenoma destruens, hydatidiform mole, maintaining remission of acute leukemia.

Dose: 15-30 mg/day × 5 days orally for choriocarcinoma.

For remission maintenance in leukemia 2.5 – 15 mg/day.

Other Uses: Rheumatoid arthritis, psoriasis, as immunosuppressants.

Available as 2.5 mg tab; 50 mg/2 ml injection.

TRADE NAME: NEOTREXATE.

Folinic acid is given simultaneously to overcome its toxicity.

METHYL CELLULOSE

Listed in Indian essential medicine list.

It is used as bulk purgative. It is semi synthetic colloidal hydrophilic derivative of cellulose water should be taken generously.

Dose: 4-6 gm/day.

It also acts as non-specific adsorbants and anti-diarrhoeal for IBS patient.

It is also used as nasal drops and contact lens solution.

METHYL DOPA

Enlisted in WHO essential medicine list.

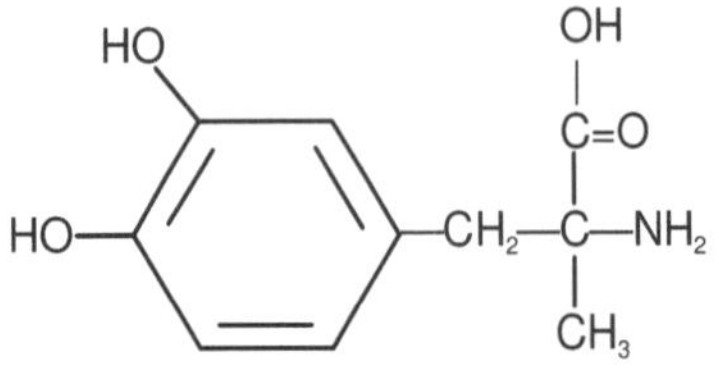

It is α methyl analogue of dopa, the precursor of dopamine and noradrenaline list used as anti-hypertensive. Methyl dopa which reduces sympathetic tone by central action is also useful for vasospastic disorders but dose requirement is high.

It is transported by intestinal amino acid transporter, less than 1/3rd of oral dose is absorbed, partly metabolized and partly excreted unchanged in urine. Anti-hypertensive effect starts after 4-6 hours and lasts about 12-24 hours.

ADR: Sedation, lethargy, reduced mental capacity, dryness of mouth, headache, nasal stuffiness, fluid retention, weight gain, impotence, positive Coomb's test, hemolytic anemia, fever, rash, hepatitis lupus syndromes, rebound hypertension on withdrawl. Its action is blocked by tricyclic anti-depressants.

Dose: 0.25 g to 5 g BD to QD.

Available as 250 mg tab.

TRADE NAME: EMDOPA; ALPHADOPA.

METHYL ERGOMETRINE

Enlisted in Indian essential medicine list.

i. This ergot preparation is used to control and prevent PPH.
ii. Caesarean section.
iii. Instrumental delivery to prevent uterine atony.
iv. To ensure normal involution.

Available as 0.125 mg tab 0.2 mg/ml injection.

Dose: For P.P.H., prevention: 0.2 to 0.3 mg I.M. in active PPH 0.5 mg I.V. for involution 0.125 mg TDS × 7 days.

TRADE NAME: METHERGIN.

METHYL PREDNISOLONE

Enlisted in Indian essential medicine list.

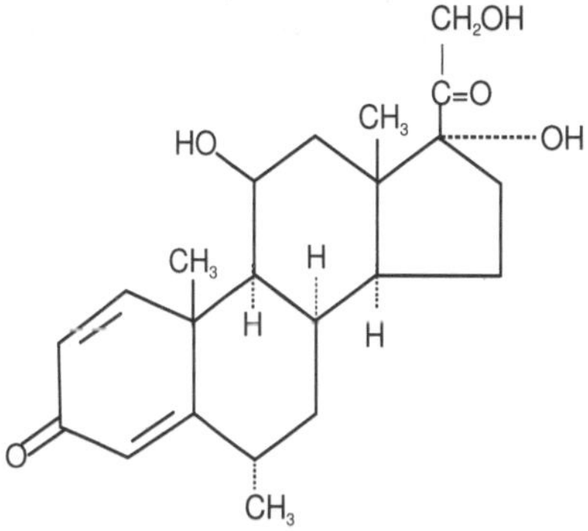

This methyl derivative of prednisolone has same actions and uses of the parent compound. It is slightly more potent than prednisolone.

Dose: 4-32 mg/day orally.

Methyl prednisolone acetate is also used as retention enema and as a pulse therapy in high dose 1 g I.V. every 6-8 weeks used in rheumatoid arthritis, renal transplant, pemphigus.

Available as 40 mg, 125 mg, 0.5 g (8 ml) and 1 g (16 ml) Inj for I.M. or I.V. use, Tablets of 2, 4, 16 mg strength.

TRADE NAME: MEDROL; SOLU-MEDROL.

METHYLTHIONINIUM CHLORIDE (METHYLENE BLUE)

Enlisted both in WHO and Indian essential medicine list.

It is dark greenish crystalline powder with a metallic lusture, hygroscopic. It is soluble in water in small doses facilitate conversion of methemoglobin to hemoglobin, so used in:

i. Cyanide poisoning.
ii. Drug induced methemoglobinemia.

Dose: 1% solution is given I.V. 1-4 mg/kg body weight. It is also used in idiopathic methemoglobinemia. Dose 300 mg orally daily with ascorbic acid (large amounts).

METOCLOPRAMIDE

WHO and Indian essential medicine enlisted drug. Chemically it is substituted benzamides.

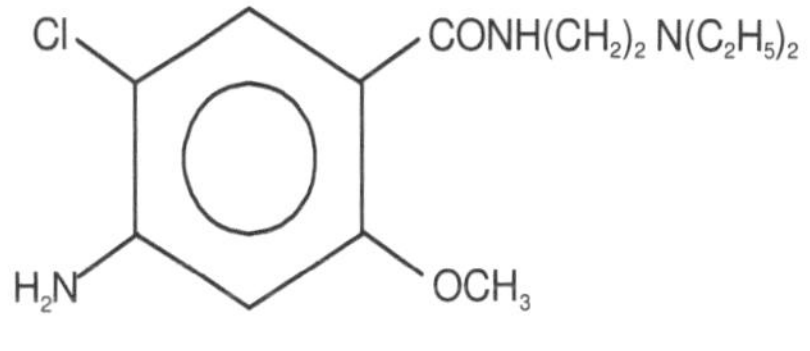

Its mechanism of action involves $5HT_4$ receptor agonism, vagal and central $5HT_3$ antagonism, possible sensitization of muscarinic receptor on smooth muscle and dopamine receptor antagonism. It is a prokinetic drug.

It is rapidly absorbed orally, enters brain, placenta and milk, conjugated in liver and excreted with urine within 24 hours. Action on oral route starts within ½ -1 hour within 10 minutes after I.M. and within 2 minutes if given I.V. and it lasts 4-6 hours.

ADR: Well tolerated but sedation, loose stool, dizziness, dystonia of muscles, galactorrhoea, gynaecomastia. Parkinsonism on prolong use may occur.

Therapeutic Uses:

i. Antiemetic.
ii. Gastrokinetics.
iii. Dyspepsia.
iv. Gastroesophageal reflux disease (GERD).

Dose: 10 mg, Children 0.2–0.5 mg/kg TDS oral or I.M. In chemotherapy induced vomiting 0.3 – 1 mg/kg slow I.V. or I.M.

Available as: 10 mg tab, 5 mg/5 ml syrup, 10 mg/2 ml injection. TRADE NAME: PERINORM; REGLAN; MAXERON.

METOPROLOL

Enlisted in Indian essential medicine list.

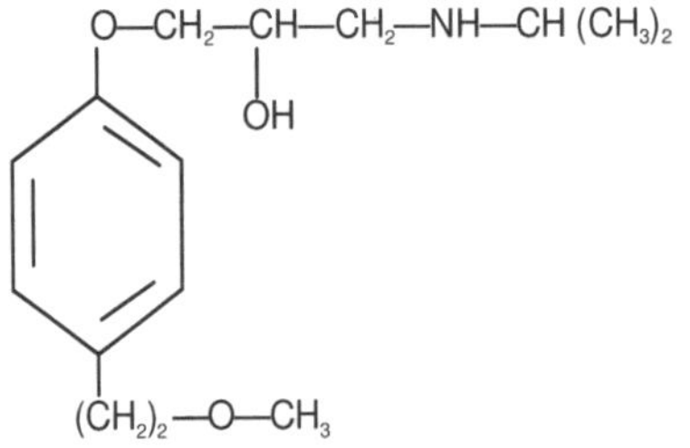

It is second generation β_1 selective blocker. It is less likely to produce asthma and may be preferred in diabetics getting insulin or OHG.

Its first pass metabolism is less. More than 90% metabolized before excretion. Dose adjustment required for slow or fast hydroxylator.

S(-) Metoprolol enantiomer is now available where dose requirement is half.

Available as 25, 50, 100 mg tab; 5 mg/ml injection.

Dose: Once daily 100-400 mg.

Therapeutic Uses: Hypertension, Ischaemic heart disease.
TRADE NAME: BETALOC; METOLAR.

METRONIDAZOLE

Enlisted both in WHO and Indian essential medicine lists.

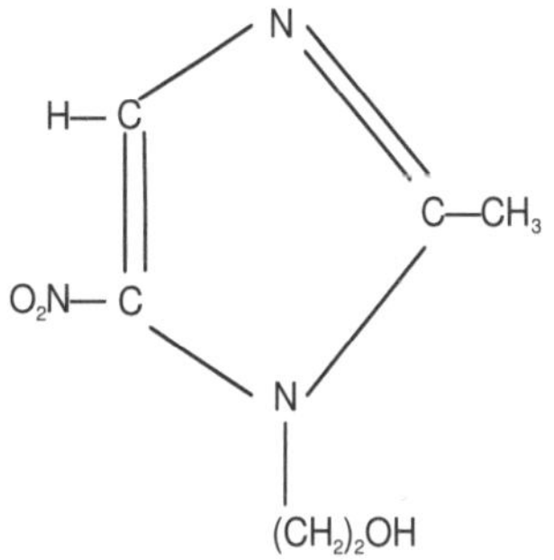

This is nitroimidazole derivative introduced for treatment of trichomoniasis but later its effect on amoeba was established. Apart from these two it is also effective against giardia anaerobic bacteria such as *Bact fragilis, Fusobacterium, Cl perfringens. Cl difficile, H.pylori, Campylobacter, Spirochetes, Anaerobic streptococci.* It facilitates extraction of Dracunculus medinesis. It is selectively toxic to anaerobic microorganism.

It is absorbed from small intestine, widely distributed in body. Metabolized by oxidation and glucuronide conjugation in liver.

ADR: Anorexia, metallic taste, abdominal cramps, loose stool, headache, glossitis, dryness of mouth, dizziness, rash, neutropenia, seizure, peripheral neuropathy. Thrombophlebites if given I.V.

It should not be given to neurological diseases, blood dyscrasia, 1st trimester of pregnancy, in alcoholics.

It produces antabuse reactions. Enzyme inducer (Rifampicin and Phenobarbitone) reduce its therapeutic effects.

Therapeutic Uses:

i. Amoebiasis.
ii. Giardiasis.
iii. Trichomonas vaginitis.
iv. Anaerobic bacterial infection.
v. Pseudomembranous enterocolitis.
vi. Peptic ulcer due to H. pylori.
vii. Guinea worm infestations.

Dose: 200-800 mg TDS varies with types of infections. 30-50 mg/kg/day × 7-10 days.

Preparations Available: 200 mg, 400 mg tabs, 200 mg/5 ml syrup, 500 mg/100 ml I.V.
TRADE NAME: FLAGYL; METROGYL; METRON; ARISTROGYL.

MEXILETINE

Enlisted in Indian essential medicine list.

It is class IB cardiac anti-arrhythmic drug can be given orally or I.V. It reduces automaticity of Purkinje fibre. It converts one way block to two way block.

Orally absorbed, metabolized in liver and excreted with urine.

ADR: Bradycardia, hypotension, A.V. block, tremor, nausea, vomiting, dizziness, confusion, blurred vision.

Dose: 100-200 mg I.V. over 10 minutes, 1 mg/min infusion. Oral 150-200 mg TDS with meals.

Therapeutic Uses: Ventricular arrhythmia after M.I. orally for ventricular extrasystole and ventricular tachycardia.

Available as 50,150 mg caps; 250 mg /10 ml infusion.
TRADE NAME: MEXITIL.

MICONAZOLE

WHO and Indian essential medicine enlisted drug.

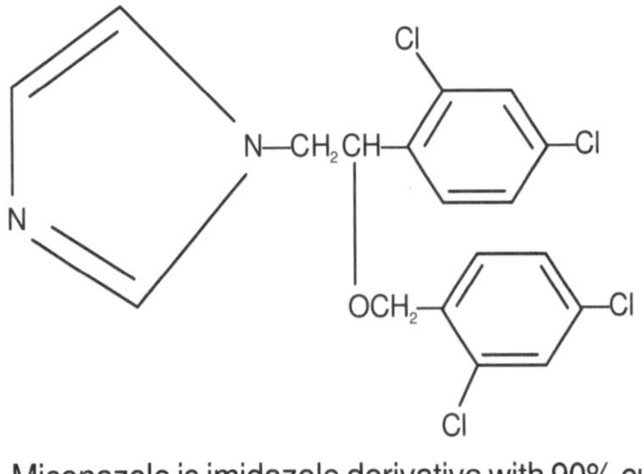

Miconazole is imidazole derivative with 90% cure rate for *Tinea, Pityriasis versicolor,* cutaneous and vaginal candidiasis, onchomycosis (because its penetrating power is good). Once application on skin acts for fews days.

ADR: Rarely, there is irritation, vaginal irritation and pelvic cramps.

Available as 2% gel; 2% vaginal gel; 2% oint; 2% lotion, dusting powder; 1% ear drops and 100 mg vaginal ovules.
TRADE NAME: DACTARIN; ZOLE.

MIDAZOLAM

Enlisted in Indian essential medicine list.

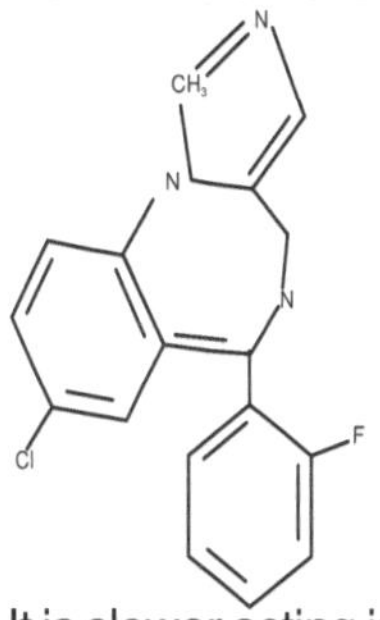

It is slower acting intravenously used benzodiazepines, used for slow acting general anaesthetics.

Midazolam is water soluble, non irritating to veins, preferred over diazepam for anaesthetic use.

Dose: 1-2.5 mg I.V.1/4th. It is also used for sedation of mechanically ventilated patients and critical care anaesthesia. Dose 0.02-0.1mg per kg / hour I.V. continuously.

Available as 1 mg/ml 5 mg/ml injection.

TRADE NAME: MEZOLAM; FULSED.

MIFEPRISTONE

Enlisted in WHO and Indian essential medicine list.

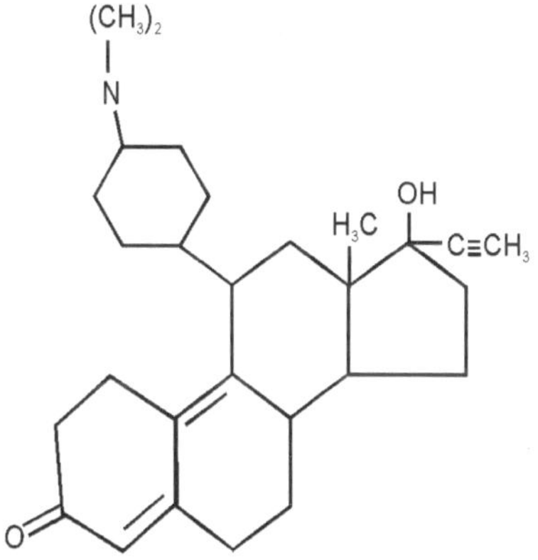

This 19 nor steroid binds strongly to progesterone receptor and inhibits its activity. It has got luteolytic property when given in midluteal period. It has anti-glucocorticoid, antiandrogenic activity. In the absence of progesterone (anovulatory cycle or after menopause), it exerts weak progestational action.

It is orally active, metabolized in liver by CYP3A4 and excreted with bile with some enterohepatic circulation.

Therapeutically Used for:

i. Termination of pregnancy.
ii. Cervical softening to attempt surgical abortion.
iii. Post coital contraceptive.
iv. Once a month contraceptive. A single dose of mifepristone 2 days after midcycle each month prevents conceptions in most of the cases.
v. Induction of labour.
vi. Cushing's syndrome inoperable cases.

Available as 200 mg tab.

TRADE NAME: MIFEPRIN; MIFEGEST.

MITOMYCIN–C

Enlisted in Indian essential medicine list.

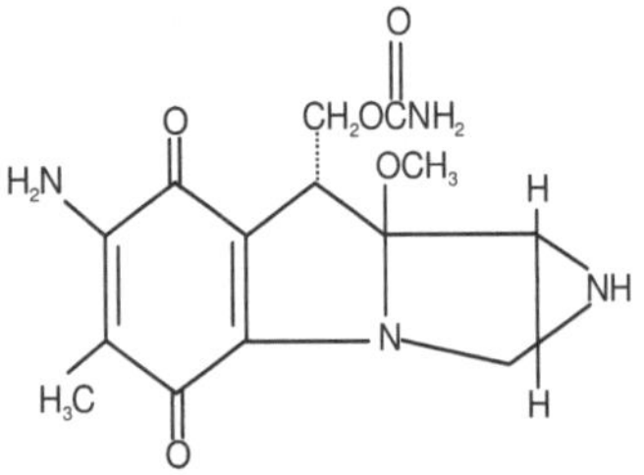

It is isolated from broth of *Streptomyces caespitosus* and has been shown to have anti-neoplastic activity. This is an alkylating agent, undergoes metabolic activation to produce its action on all phases of cell cycle. It is best drug to attack hypoxic tumour cells.

ADR: Bon marrow depression, mucositis, nausea are major ADR.

Therapeutic Uses: Resistant cancer of stomach, cervix, colon, rectum, bladder.

Available as 2, 10 mg/inj.

Dose: 10 mg/squaremeter, body surface area I.V. in one day or divided into five days.

TRADE NAME: MITOMYCIN-C.

MORPHINE

Enlisted both in WHO and Indian essential medicine list.

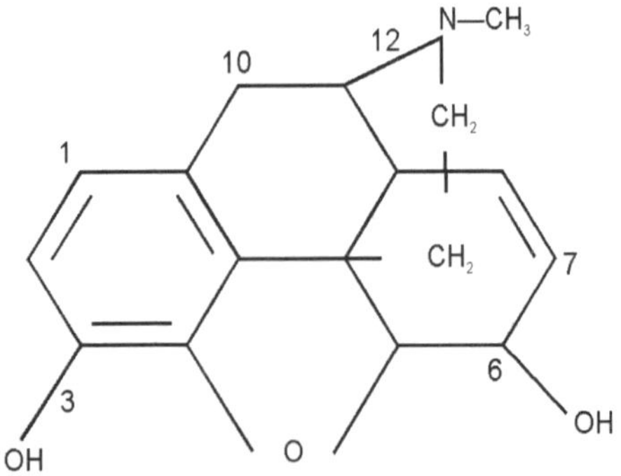

This alkaloid is phenanthrene derivative, obtained from resinous, material obtained from poppy *(Papaver somniferum)* capsules.

Its oral absorption is unreliable because of high first pass metabolism. It is 30% protein bound, concentration in liver, kidney and spleen are higher than plasma. Crosses placenta, metabolized by glucuronide conjugation. Morphine 6-glucuronide is active metabolite accumulates during chronic dosing.

ADR: Sedation, mental clouding, lethargy, respiratory depression, urinary retention, blurred vision, hypotension, urticaria, itch, swelling of lips, apnoea in newborn, tolerance and dependence.

Treatment of Morphine Poisoning:

i. Respiratory support.
ii. Gastric lavage with potassium permanganate.
iii. Antidote naloxone 0.4-0.8 mg I.V. to be repeated every 2-3 minutes till respiration picks up.

Signs of morphine poisoning are: Stupor, coma, pin point pupil, shallow respiration, cyanosis, hypotension, convulsion, pulmonary edema and respiratory failure at last.

Treatment of morphine tolerance: Substitute morphine with oral methadone and gradually withdrawing it also.

Therapeutic Uses of Morphine:

i. Analgesics.
ii. Preanaesthetic medications.
iii. Balanced anaesthesia and surgical analgesia.
iv. LVF.
v. Relief of anxiety and apprehension.
vi. Cough.
vii. Diarrhoea.

Contraindication and Precautions of Morphine Use

i. Infants and elderly.
ii. Asthma and COPD, corpulmonale, pulmonary fibrosis.
iii. Head injury.
iv. Hypotensive state.
v. Undiagnosed acute abdomen.
vi. Hypothyroid.
vii. Unstable personalities.

Dose: 10-50 mg oral, 10-15 mg I.M. or S.C. or 2-6 mg I.V., 2-3 mg epidural, intrathecal; children 0.1-0.2 mg/kg.

Available as 10, 30, 60, 100 mg continuous release tablets 10 mg/ml injection.

TRADE NAME: MORPHINE SULPHATE; MORCONTIN.

MULTIVITAMINS

Enlisted in Indian essential medicine list.

Prophylactic multivitamins should contain half to one and half times the recommended dietary allowances except for vitamin D which should not exceed the daily allowances. It may contain 4-5 times of the recommended daily allowances. Selective vitamin B factor deficiency occurs rarely, so combined therapy is required. While prescribing multivitamins, other drugs prescribed should be kept in mind viz vit B_6 may interfere Parkinsonism.

It generally acts as placebo and should be used only in deficiency states or when there is increased demand.

MUMPS VACCINE

WHO enlisted essential medicine.

Prepared from mumps virus grown in cell culture of chick embryo. A single dose generally gives protection for 10 years. Revaccination is not required. Clinical disease may occur if the vaccine is given after exposure to natural mumps. Its combination vaccine with measles and rubella is also available.

NALIDIXIC ACID

Enlisted in Indian essential medicine list.

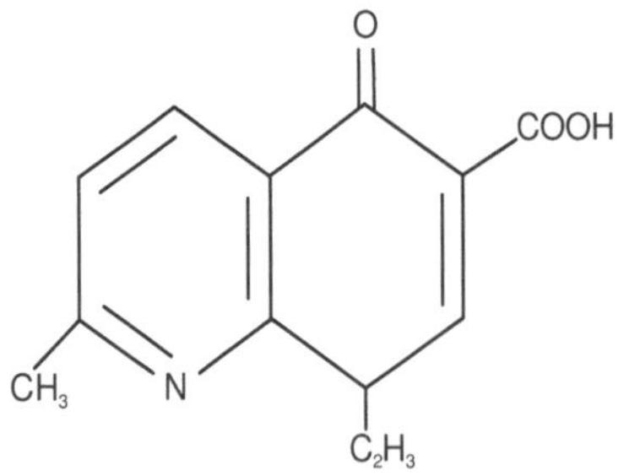

Its spectrum includes gram negative bacteria especially coliforms *E coli, Klebsiella, Enterobacter, Shigella, Pseudomonas.* It is bacteriocidal inhibits DNA gyrase.

It is orally absorbed, protein bound, partly metabolized and excreted with urine. It attains higher concentration in urine.

ADR: G.I. upset, rash, headache, drowsiness, vertigo, visual disturbance, seizure, phototoxicity (rarely), haemolysis with glucose G-pO_4ase deficiency patient. It should not be given to infants.

Dose: 0.5-1 gm TDS or QDS.

Available as 0.5 mg tab; 0.3 g/5 ml syrup.

Therapeutic Uses: U.T.I., diarrhea of *Proteus, E. coli Shigella, Salmonella*, Gonorrhea.
TRADE NAME: GRAMONEG; WINTOMYLON.

NALOXONE

WHO and Indian essential medicine enlisted drug.

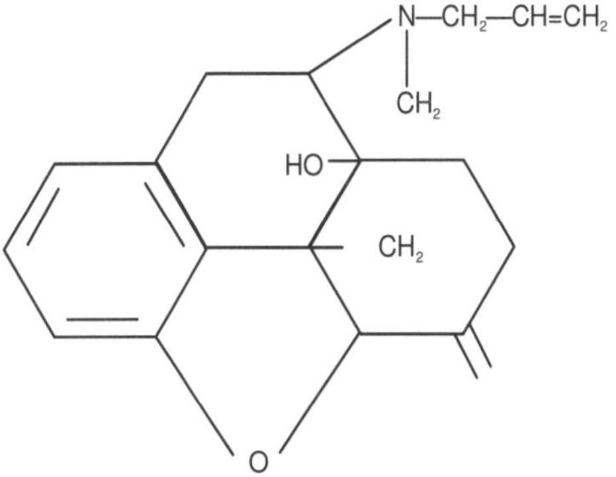

This opioid antagonist is N-alyenoroxymorphone and competes for all types of opioid receptors and devoid of any type of agonistic action even at higher doses.

Given 0.4-0.8 mg I.V. it antagonizes all actions of morphine. It precipitates morphine withdrawl also. It also blocks endogenous opioid peptides and blocks placebo, acupuncture and stress induced analgesia.

It is inactive orally because of high first pass metabolism, metabolized by glucuronidation.

ADR: Rare; rise of BP and pulmonary edema may occur.

Therapeutic Uses:

i. Morphine poisoning 0.4-0.8 mg I.V. every 2-3 min.
ii. For reversing neonatal asphyxia if mother received opioid during labour.
iii. To diagnose opioid dependence (will precipitate withdrawl).
iv. Raises BP in shock and spinal injury patient.

Available as 0.4 mg /ml (adult) and 0.04 mg/2 ml (infants ampoules).
TRADE NAME: NORCONTAN; NALOX.

NELFINAVIR (NVF)

WHO and Indian essential medicine enlisted drug.

This is retroviral protease inhibitor effective against HIV. Its absorption is higher in fed state. It is metabolized by CYP3A and excreted with faeces.

ADR: Diarrhea, flatulance. Diarrhoea often responds to anti-diarrhoeal. It inhibits CYP3A and is involved in multiple drug interactions. If given with rifabutin its dose has to be increased. It can be given to pregnant women.

Available as 750 mg tab.

Dose: 750 mg TDS.

TRADE NAME: NELFIN; NELVIR.

NEOMYCIN

WHO enlisted essential medicine.

This aminoglycosides is obtained from *S. fradiae* active against gram negative bacilli and gram positive cocci except *Pseudomonas* and *Strepto. pyogenes.* It is highly toxic so not used systematically. Orally not absorbed. Oral and topical administrations are generally devoid of systemic toxicity. Small amount absorbed and excreted with urine.

Dose: 0.25-1gm. QID orally; 0.3-0.5% topically.

Therapeutic Uses:

i. Topically on wounds, ulcer, burns, external ear infection, conjunctivitis.
ii. Orally for bowel preparation before surgery and hepatic coma.

ADR: Rash, sensitization, malabsorption after oral ingestion, superinfection with candida.

NEOMYCIN WITH BACITRACIN

This combination is enlisted in both WHO and Indian essential medicine list.

Bacitracin is an antibiotic first discovered from bacteria *Bacillus* subtilis. It is active against gram positive cocci and bacilli. It inhibits cell wall.

Orally not absorbed, parenteral highly toxic. Used topically on wounds, ulcers, eye infection.

Not useful for furuncle, boil and carbuncle because does not penetrate intact skin.

NEOSTIGMINE

WHO and Indian essential medicine enlisted drug.

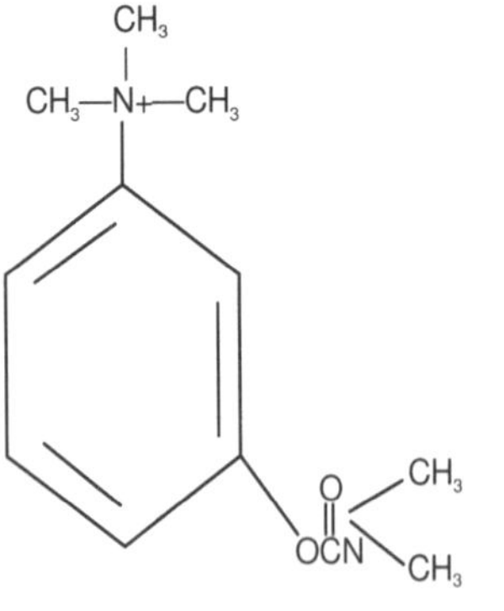

This carbamate derivative acts as reversible anti-cholinesterase.

Therapeutic Uses:

i. To terminate supraventricular tachycardia.
ii. Post operative urinary retention and G.I.T. atony.
iii. In diagnosis and treatment of myasthenia gravis.
iv. Gallamine toxicity.

ADR: Hyperhydrosis, salivation, G.I. distress, muscle cramps, weakness, fasciculation, overdose may cause cholinergic crisis.

Contraindications: Mechanical obstruction to urinary and G.I. tract, bronchial asthma, bradycardia, should not be used with choline esters or depolarizing neuromuscular blocking agents.

Available as 15 mg tab, 0.5 mg/ml in 1 and 5 ml container.
TRADE NAME: PROSTIGMINE; MYOSTIGMINE.

NEVIRAPINE

WHO and Indian essential medicine enlisted drug.

It is non-nucleoside reverse transcriptase inhibitor inhibits HIV without intracellular phosphorylation. Orally absorbed, not food dependent, lipophilic, enters CSF. t/2 25-30 hours. Metabolized by CYP3A to hydroxylated metabolites and excreted with urine. It also inhibits transmission of HIV from mother to newborn if given in the onset of labour.

Dose: 200 mg/day, may be increased to 200 mg BD.

Available as 200 mg tab.

ADR: Rash, nausea, headache, fever, rise of liver, enzymes. Avoid its use with rifampicin (enzyme inducer) or ketoconazole (enzyme inhibitors).
TRADE NAME: NEVIMUME; NEVIVIR.

NICLOSAMIDE

WHO and Indian essential medicine enlisted drug.

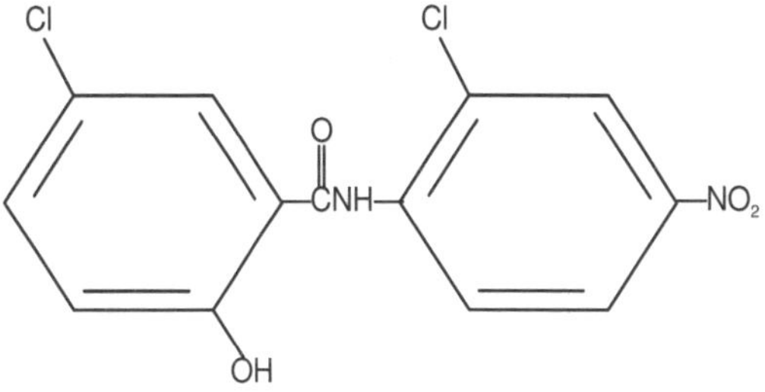

Effective against large tapeworms *T. saginata T. solium* D latum and dwarf tapeworm *H. nana*. It causes segments to disintegrate releasing viable eggs, so if taken for T. solium, a laxative should be taken within two hours to avoid possibilities of cysticercosis.

Treatment of pregnant woman may be deferred because tapeworm infestations are not life threatening.

ADR: Nausea, Malaise, Pain abdomen.

Dose: 2 tabs to be swallowed, followed by another two tablets after 1 hour and a saline purge.

Available as 0.5 g tab.

TRADE NAME: NICLOSAN.

NICOTINAMIDE

WHO and Indian essential medicine enlisted drug.

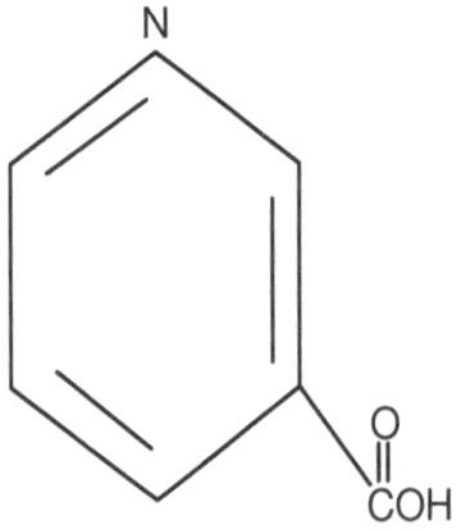

Niacin is pteridine derivative, converted to body into niacinamide, the physiological active form. It is a component of two important co-enzymes that effect tissue respiration and energy transfer in glycolysis and lipid metabolism. It is also called pellagra preventing factor. Tryptophan is regarded as provitamin, partially converted to nicotinic acid.

It is orally absorbed, metabolized and stored in liver and excreted with urine.

Deficiency produces: Dermatitis, diarrhoea, dementia, chronic alcoholics are generally sufferer.

Available as 50 mg tablet. Injection 100 mg/10 ml as nicotinic acid. Nicotinamide tab 50 mg and inj 50 mg/ml.

Dose: Therapeutic 50 to 250 mg daily; Prophylactic 15-30 mg daily.

Therapeutic Uses:

i. Prophylactic.
ii. Pellagra.
iii. Hartnup's disease.

iv. Peripheral vascular disease and hyperlipidaemia (nicotinic acid is used).

ADR: Flushing, urticaria, pruritis, furunculosis, malaise, amblyopia, hyperuricaemia, janudice, impaired glucose tolerance.

NIFEDIPINE

Enlisted both in WHO and Indian essential medicine list.

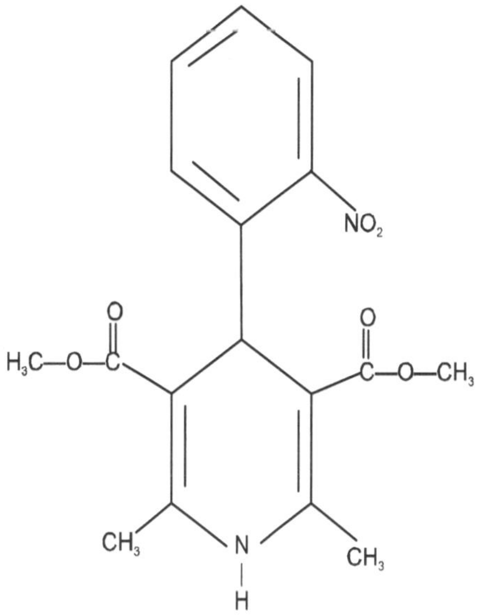

This calcium channel blocker belongs to lipophilic dihydropyridine with rapid onset and short duration of action. It causes arteriolar dilatation and decreases BP by decreasing total peripheral resistance. It has weak negative inotropic effect. It causes tachycardia due to reflex sympathetic stimulation. It has mild natriuretic action. It increases coronary flow.

It is orally absorbed, metabolized in the liver.

ADR: Palpitation, flushing, ankle edema, hypotension, headache, drowsiness, nausea. It may paradoxically increase angina. Difficulty in bladder voiding and hampers diabetic control.

Therapeutic Uses: Antihypertensive, antianginal, premature, labour, Raynaud's disease.

Available as 5, 10, 20 mg tabs.

Dose: 5-20 mg BD to TDS.

TRADE NAME: CALCIGARD; DEPIN; NICARDIA.

NITRAZEPAM

Enlisted in Indian essential medicine list.

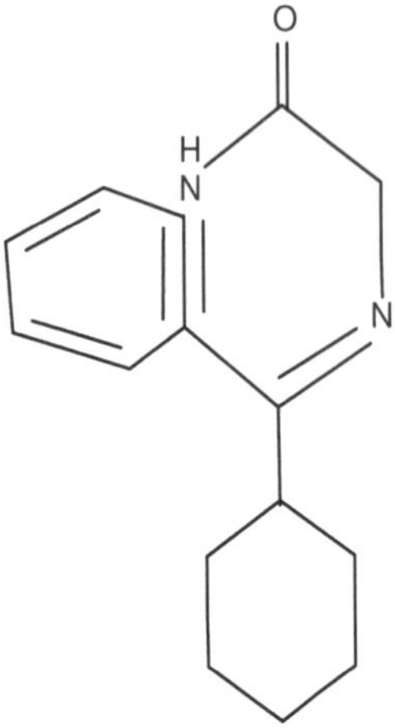

This is a benzodiazepine derivative, used as hypnotics. This drug is slowly eliminated. Long acting t/2 30 hours.

Dose for insomnia 5-10 mg.

Therapeutic Uses: Chronic insomnia, short term insomnia with anxiety, night awakening, preoperatively.

Available as 5 mg tab, 10 mg cap.

TRADE NAME: SEDAMON; HYPNOTEX.

NITROFURANTOIN

Enlisted both in WHO and Indian essential medicine list.

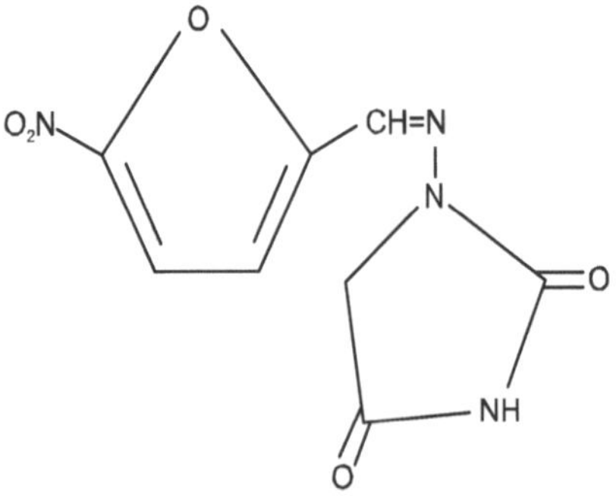

Nitrofurantoin exhibits wide spectrum of anti bacterial activity against gram positive and gram negative organisms including *E. coli, Staph pyogenes, Paracolobactrum, Enterobacter, Klebsiella, Indole positive proteins.*

It is orally absorbed from G.I.T., highly protein bound with poor tissue level, high urinary concentration. Mostly bacteriostatic.

Dose: 400-800 mg/day in 2-4 divided doses. Alkalination of urine reduces antibacterial action. It is given is full dose for 10-14 days then with smaller doses for several weeks to months. It is mainly excreted with urine by filtration and tubular secretion, so should not be used in renal insufficiency.

Nalidoxic acid antagonizes its action. It is available as 50,100 mg tab; 25 mg/5 ml suspension.
TRADE NAME: FURADANTIN.

NITROUS OXIDE

Enlisted both in WHO and Indian essential medicine list.

It is sweet smelling non explosive gas with low anaesthetic potency. Always used with 20% oxygen for induction and 34% oxygen for maintenance. It is colourless supplied in steel cylinders under pressure. It is non irritating. It is good analgesic, even 20% produces analgesia equivalent to morphine. Its muscle relaxation power is poor, so often requires neuromuscular blockers. Loss of consciousness occurs in 65-70%.

It is not altered in body and carried as physical solution in blood. It is not bound to haemoglobin and other body tissues, eliminated with lung within 2-5 minutes of withdrawl. It produces amnesia, hence called "laughing gas". It should be used in presence of witness. The oxygen of nitrous oxide molecule is not available for tissue respiration.

NORETHISTERONE

Enlisted both in WHO and Indian essential medicine list.

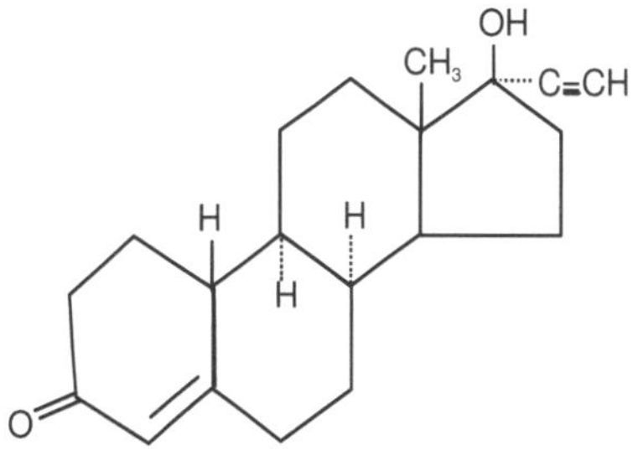

This is 19-nortestosterone derivative progesterone. Orally used in the dose of 5-10 mg OD to BD. Supplied as 1, 2 and 5 mg tab.

Therapeutic Uses:

i. Primary and secondary amenorrhoea 5-15 mg daily.
ii. DUB 10-30 mg/day.
iii. Endometriosis 20-30 mg/day.
iv. Dysmenorrhoea.
v. Premenstrual tension.
vi. O.C.P.
vii. Hormone replacement therapy.

ADR: Breast engorgement, headache, rise in body temperature, increased risk of breast cancer, lowers HDL levels and increases chances of atherogenesis and nausea.

TRADE NAME: PRIMOLUT-N.

NORFLOXACIN

Enlisted in Indian essential medicine list.

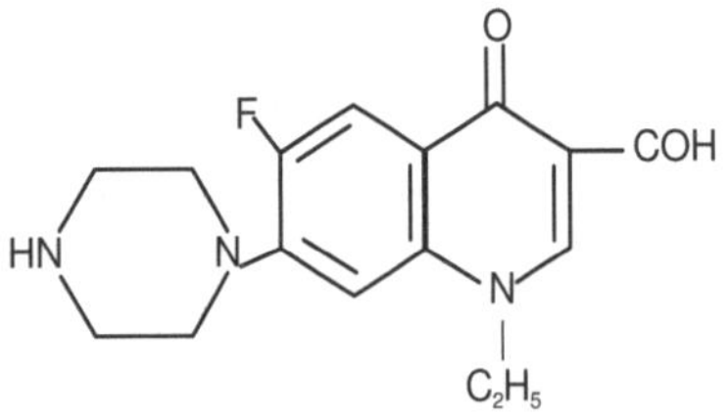

Norfloxacin is 2nd generation fluoroquinolone, less potent than ciprofloxacin. It metabolized and excreted unchanged in urine. Generally used for urogenital tract infection, diarrhoea caused by bacteria. It is ineffective in R.T.I. and other systemic infections caused by gram positive cocci.

Available as 200, 400, 800 mg tab; 3 mg/ml eye drops.

Dose: 200-400 mg BD for U.T.I.

TRADE NAME: NORBACTIN; NORFLOX.

NYSTATIN

WHO and Indian essential medicine enlisted drug.

This is polyene macrolide topically used antifungal drug (systemic use is too toxic). It is obtained from S. noursei. Not absorbed orally, so used for monilial diarrhoea due to superinfection.

Used for vaginal moniliasis, oral thrush, corneal conjunctival and cutaneous candidiasis.

ADR: Nausea, bad taste if given orally. It is not effective for dermatophytosis.

Available as 5 lac U tab; 1 lac U vaginal tab; 1 lac U/gram ointment.

TRADE NAME: MICOSTATIN.

OFLOXACIN

Ofloxacin is a fluoroquinolone (FQ). It inhibits the bacterial enzyme DNA gyrase. It is active against gram positive, gram negative, anaerobes, chlamydia, mycoplasma.

Used for urethritis, cervicitis, atypical pneumonia, *M. tuberculosis, M. leprae,* bronchitis, ENT infection, gonorrhoea.

It is lipid soluble, orally absorbed. Its absorption is not interfered by food, excreted mostly unchanged in urine. Inhibition of theophyllin metabolism is less compared to other (FQS).

Available as 100, 200, 400 mg tab; 200 mg/100 ml I.V. infusion, 50 mg/5 ml suspension; 0.3% eye drop.

OMEPRAZOLE

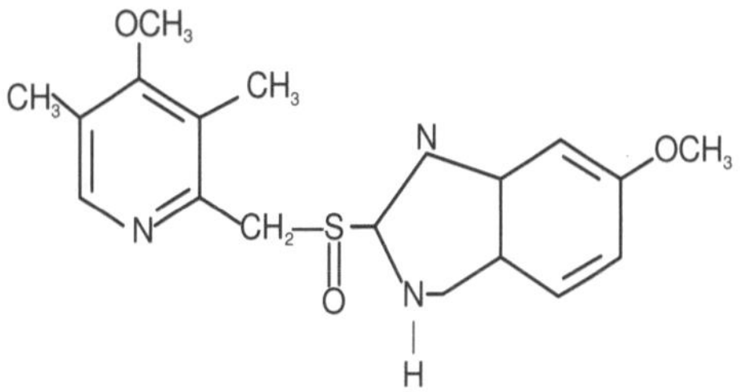

It is a proton pump inhibitor (PPI), chemically substituted benzimidazole, inhibits final common step of gastric acid secretion. It is inactive in neutral pH but active below pH of 5. It is tightly bound to $H^{\pm}K^{+}$ATPase pump. It is a hit and run drug, acid secretion of parietal cells restarts when new $H^{+}K^{+}$ ATPase molecules are synthesized. It also inhibits carbonic anhydrase of gastric mucosa.

Orally 50% absorbed, bioavailability is reduced by food, so taken in empty stomach. Plasma protein bound, metabolized by CYP2C19 of liver and metabolic products are excreted in urine. Compensatory hypergastrinaemia may occur. No dose adjustment required for elderly or for liver and kidney impaired patient.

Available as 20 and 40 mg caps or enteric coated granules.

Nausea, loose motion, headache, joint pain, dizziness, rash, atropic gastritis on prolong use. It inhibits the metabolism of phenytoin, diazepam. Its metabolism is inhibited by clarithromycin.

Therapeutic Uses: Peptic ulcer, gastro-oesophageal reflux diseases, Zollinger-Ellison syndrome, aspiration pneumonia.

ONDANSETRON

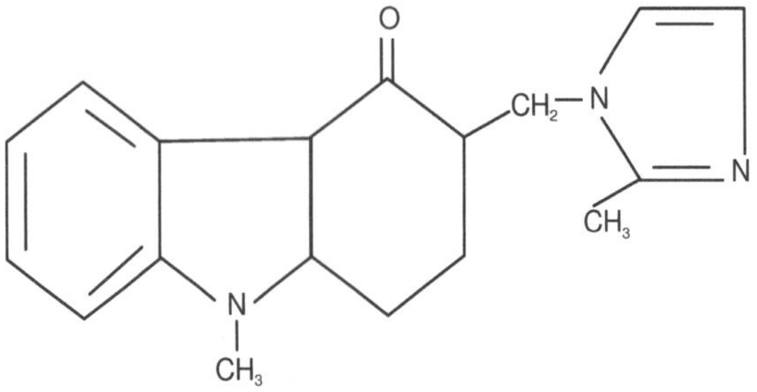

Ondansetron is selective $5HT_3$ receptor antagonist. Generally used to control chemotherapy, radiotherapy, post operative nausea and vomiting. It blocks vomiting impulses at peripheral and central relay.

It is orally absorbed, hydroxylated by $CYPIA_2$ eliminated by urine and faeces.

Available as 4, 8 mg tabs; 2 mg/ml in 2 ml and 4 ml ampoules.

ADR: Headache, constipation, diarrhea, abdominal discomfort, rashes may occur after I.V. injection.

ORAL POLIOMYELITIS VACCINE (Live Attenuated)

It is live attenuated virus (Polio virus 1, 2, 3) grown in monkey kidney cell culture available as 10 ml and 50 ml vials.

Dose is 2 drops directly in mouth.

Virus grows in intestines and produces immunity. It is a component of universal immunization programme given at birth, 6, 10, 14 weeks and booster in 15-18 months and at school entry. Simultaneously given to all children below 5 years is called Pulse Polio Programme.

It is advisable to postpone the vaccination if child is suffering vomiting or diarrhoea. Paralysis due to vaccination may occur but is extremely rare.

ORAL REHYDRATION SALT (O.R.S.)

In diarrhoea and vomiting treatment of fluid and electrolyte loss is important. It can be done with O.R.S. or I.V. fluid administration.

WHO formula of ORS (New)

NaCl	2.6 gm
KCl	1.5 gm
Tri-sodium citrate	2.9 gm

Glucose	13.5 gm
Water	1 litre
Total osmolarity	245 mOSm/L

Non Diarrhoeal Use of QRS

i. Post burn, post surgical, post trauma maintenance of hydration.
ii. Heat stroke.

OXAMNIQUINE

This drug is enlisted in WHO essential medicine list.

It is semi-synthetic tetrahydroquinoline. Orally absorbed, used for *S. mansoni.*

Dose: 10-15 mg/kg once.

Dizziness, headache, drowsiness, vomiting, diarrhoea, colic, pruritis, urticaria, driving should be avoided for 24 hours because of drowsiness.

Available as 250 mg cap; 50 mg/ml susp.

OXYTOCIN

Oxytocin is a nonapeptide secreted by posterior pituitary.

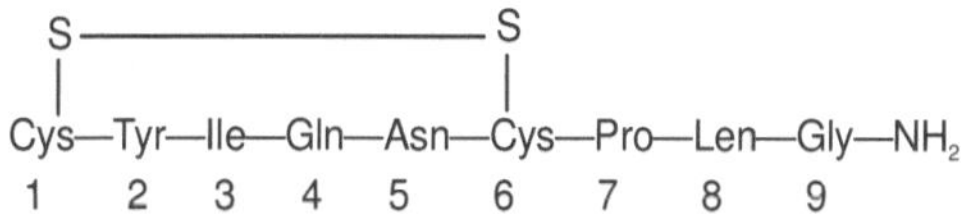

It acts on myometrium of uterus on oxytocin receptors the number of which increases in later part of pregnancy. It has physiologic role in labour, millk ejection reflex and it acts as peptide neurotransmitter of brainstem and hypothalamus.

Since it is peptide, has to be given by I.M. or I.V. or rarely intranasal spray. It is degraded by liver and kidney. Pregnant woman elaborate oxytocinase. Standardization 1 I.U. oxytocin 2 microgram pure hormone.

Available as 2 I.U./2 ml or 5 I.U./ml inj.

Therapeutic Uses:

i. Induction of labour (5 I.U. slow I.V. with 500 ml of glucose).
ii. Uterine inertia.
iii. Postpartum haemorrhage.
iv. Breast engorgement given as intranasal spray.
v. Oxygen challenge test to determine utero placental insufficiency, will raise foetal heart rate markedly.

OXYGEN

Oxygen gas is essential for human survival.

Oxygen I.P. is dispensed in compressed cylinder painted black with white shoulder.

Therapeutic Uses:

i. Hypoxia.
ii. Alveolar hypoventilation.
iii. Ventilation in excess of perfusion as in anaesthesia.
iv. Intrapulmonary shunting of blood.
v. Venous admixture of blood.
vi. Right to left cardiac shunt.
vii. Decreased central venous oxygen content.

HYPERBARIC OXYGEN is used for:

i. Respiratory disease of newborn.
ii. Carbon monoxide poisoning.
iii. Decompression sickness.
iv. Anaerobic infection.
v. Surgery (open heart).
vi. Circulatory disturbances.
vii. To make malignant cells radiosensitive.

Adverse Effects of Oxygen Therapy:

i. May damage pulmonary epithelium if used for prolonged period.
ii. C.N.S. : Paresthesia, twitching, convulsion, loss of consciousness.
iii. Carbondioxide narcosis.
iv. Fire hazard.
v. Retrolental fibroplasia with hyperbaric oxygen.

PACLITAXEL

Enlisted in essential medicine list of India.

This anticancer is taxanes, obtained from alkaloid ester derived from Yews of Pacific (*Taxus brevifolia*) and Yews of Europe (Taxus buccata). The alkaloid from it has high affinity for binding microtubules and enhances the tubulin polymerization that is it is mitotic spindle poison.

Therapeutic Uses: Solid tumor *viz* ovarian advanced breast, small and non small cell lungs, prostrate, head and neck oesophagus, bladder, Kaposi's sarcoma.

Given by I.V. route metabolized extensively by liver and excreted with feces. Hypersensitivity reaction can be reduced by prior administration of dexamethasone.

ADR: Bone marrow depression, peripheral neuropathy, chest pain, arthralgia, myalgia, mucositis, oedema.

Dose: 130-170 mg sq mt I.V. over 3 to 24 hours every 3-4 weeks.

Abraxane is paclitaxel which is albumin bound does not produce hypersensitivity reaction.

Available as 30 mg in 5 ml cremophor emulsion (Polyoxyethylated castor oil + alcohol + water per vial). The hypersensitivity reaction is due to cremophor solvent.

TRADE NAME: INTAXEL; PAXTAL.

PANCURONIUM

Enlisted in essential medicine list of India.

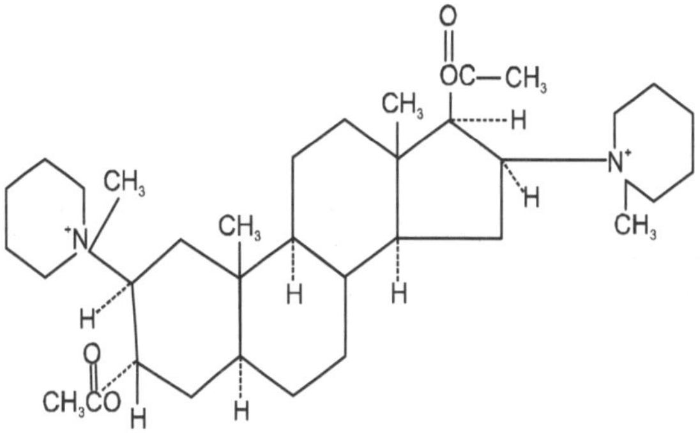

This synthetic steroid, non depolarizing, competitive blocker is acting as neuromuscular relaxant. It is 5 times more potent than d-tubocurarine. Other advantages are good cardiovascular stability due to less ganglion blockade, less flushing, bronchospasm or cardiac arrhythmia due to less histamine release. BP may rise due to vagal blockade. Eliminated by kidneys. Requires reversal. Used for long time requiring operations like neurosurgery.

Available as 2 mg/ml in 2 ml ampoules.

TRADE NAME: PAVULON; NEOCURON.

PARACETAMOL

Enlisted in WHO and Indian essential medicine list.

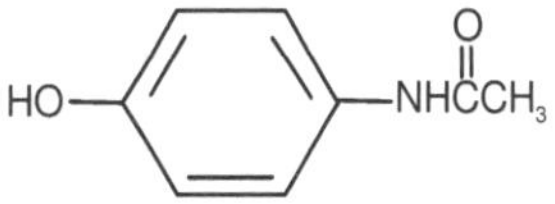

This analgesic and antipyretic is a NSAID metabolic, product of phenacetin and acetanilide used for headache, mild myalgia, arthralgia fever. It produces little or methemoglobinemia and hemolytic anemia. It is more active in cox of brain.

Orally absorbed, 25% protein bound, uniformly distributed, metabolized by conjugation with glucuronic acid and sulfate and excreted with urine.

ADR: Nausea, rash, nephropathy on heavy ingestion (Papillary necrosis, tubular atrophy, renal fibrosis). Acute poisoning occurs if taken more than 150 mg/kg or more than 10 gm. Hepatic necrosis, tubular necrosis, hypoglycemia causing hepatic failure. It occurs due to N-acetyl–p-benzoquinoneimine (NABQI) production by paracetamol which is detoxified by conjugation with glutathione so it is binding to protein of liver and kidney proteins causing their necrosis. Toxicity is more with alcoholics.

Treated by N-acetylcysteine 150 mg/kg over 15 min and to repeat after 20 hours. It may be given orally 75 mg/kg every 4-6 hours (MUCOMIX 300 mg/ml in 2 and 5 ml container) which replenishes the depleted glutathione. Other supportive measures plus gastric lavage with activated charcoal should be done.

Available as: 05, 1 g tab, 125 mg/5 ml syrup, 150 mg/ml drops, 300 mg/2 ml injection.

TRADE NAME: CROCIN; PYRIGESIC; FEBRINIL.

PAROMOMYCIN

WHO enlisted essential medicine list.

This is an aminoglycoside used orally to treat diarrhoea of enteropathogenic *E. coli* though other aminoglycosides are preferred. Other uses are amoebocidal, since it suppresses the gut flora and hence decreases bacteria production of NH_3, so used in hepatic coma. It is also effective against *T. saginata; T. solium; D. latum, H. nana.*

ADR: Nausea, diarrhoea, rash, vertigo, abdominal pain, vomiting, oto and nephrotoxicity. Poorly absorbed and almost all drug is eliminated with stool.

Dose: 25 mg/kg in divided doses × 5 days.

Available as 250 mg cap.

TRADE NAME: HUMATIN.

PENICILLAMINE

This essential medicine is enlisted both in WHO and Indian essential medicine list.

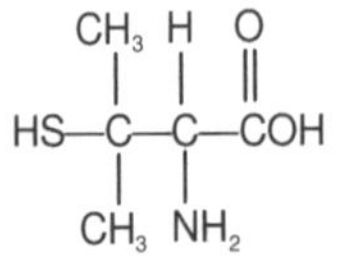

This is a synthetic preparation originally derived from degradation of penicillin, without any antibacterial effect, marketed as D-isomer. L-isomer produces optic neuritis.

Chelates: Cu, Fe, Pb and probably other heavy metals with which it forms soluble complex which is excreted with urine. It is orally effective.

Therapeutic Uses:

i. Wilson's disease (hepatolenticular degeneration) (life long therapy).
ii. Cu and Hg poisoning.
iii. Pb poisoning.
iv. Cystinurea since it promotes cysteine excretion.
v. Scleroderma benefits by increasing soluble collagen.
vi. Rheumatoid arthritis as disease modifying drug.

ADR: Cutaneous reaction, itching, fever, may occur with short term therapy for metal poisoning treatment. Long term treatment produces dermatological, renal, hematological and collagen tissue toxicities.

Available as 150, 250 mg caps.

Dose: 0.5 to 1 g daily in divided doses 1 hours before, 2 hours after meal to avoid chelation of foods, heavy metals.

TRADE NAME: ARTAMIN; ARTIN; CILAMIN.

PENTAMIDINE ISOTHIONATE

Enlisted both in WHO and Indian essential medicine list.

This diamidine is active against *L. donovani, Trypanosomes, Pneumocystis jovoveci,* some bacteria and fungi. It probably acts with kinetoplast DNA to inhibit topoisomerase II or interferes with aerobic glycolysis.

Dose: 4 mg/kg deep IM or slow IV on alternate days 5-15 weeks, to be repeated after 2 weeks. After absorption from injection site it is taken up by tissues, liver, kidney and stored for months.

ADR: Hypoglycemia due to cytolysis of β cells of pancreas, headache, fever, rigor, hypotension, collapse, angioedema due to histamine release.

Supplied by 200 and 300 mg (lomidine) by Govt agencies. The dry powder of vials should be dissolved to yield 10% solution before injection.

PENTAZOCINE

Indian essential medicine enlisted drug.

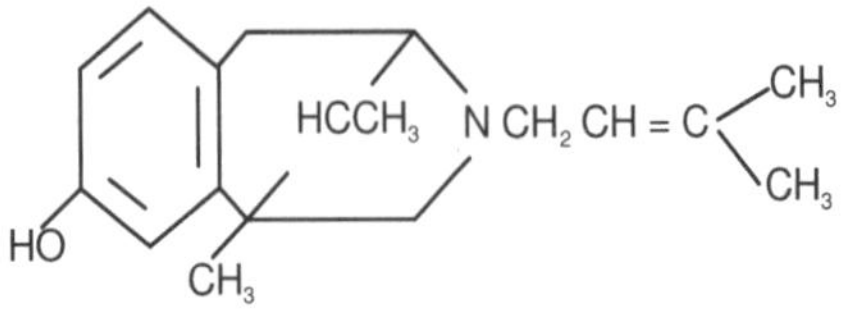

This is an analgesic narcotic of benzomorphane series. It is also a weak narcotic antagonist. It is (agonist to kappa receptor and antagonism to MU receptor). It is effective in relieving pain of moderate nature (obstetrics) though it can cause foetal respiratory depression. It does not have anti-inflammatory effect.

Orally absorbed, though considerable first pass effect occurs oral to perenteral ratio is 1:1. It is oxidized and glucuronide conjugate and excreted with urine.

Dose: 50-100 mg daily orally, 30-60 mg I.M. or subcutaneous local injection may cause fibrosis.

ADR: Nausea, vomiting, dizziness, euphoria, diaphoresis, constipation, urinary retentions, transient hypertension, biliary spasm, tolerance, physical dependence, withdrawl symptoms.

Available as 25 mg tab, 30 mg/ml injection.

Therapeutic Uses: Post operative pain, burn, trauma, fracture, cancer pain.

PERMETHRIN

WHO enlisted essential medicine.

This potent broad spectrum pyrethoid insecticide used for scabies and lice to which it causes paralysis by delaying depolarization. It persists on skin for days after application and its systemic absorption is low and its resistance is also very low.

ADR: Tingling, burning, itching, rash, erythema.

Available as 5% cream, 1% soap, 5% lotion. It is first choice drug for pediculosis and scabies.

For scabies 5% cream applied all over the body except face and head and wash after 8-12 hours; for lice 1% lotion applied over scalp and washed after 10 minutes.

TRADE NAME: PERMITE; PERLICE.

PERTUSSIS VACCINE

Enlisted in WHO essential medicine list.

Immunization against pertussis is strongly recommended because the disease is highly communicable and responsible for majority of deaths below 1 year of age. Pertussis has decreased in last 40 years because of widespread use of vaccines. Generally it is given with diphtheria and tetanus toxoids.

Pertussis vaccine is used instead of DPT if infants have shown neurological complications with DPT to complete the series. It is killed 2×10^{10} organisms/ml suspension of *B pertussis* organism.

Dose: 0.25- 0.5 ml subcutaneous or I.M. at monthly intervals below 5 years of age (pertussis is rare after 5 years). It also induces decreased beta adrenergic activity and helps in the sensitization of other antigens.

Convulsion in infants following DPT is believed to be due to pertussis components. Other ADR local pain, induration, high fever, convulsion, altered consciousness, focal neurological signs may occur. Any of such reaction is contraindiction of its use. Other contraindications are convulsions and neurological diseases.

Now-a-days it is rarely used separately.

PETHIDINE

Enlisted in Indian essential medicine list.

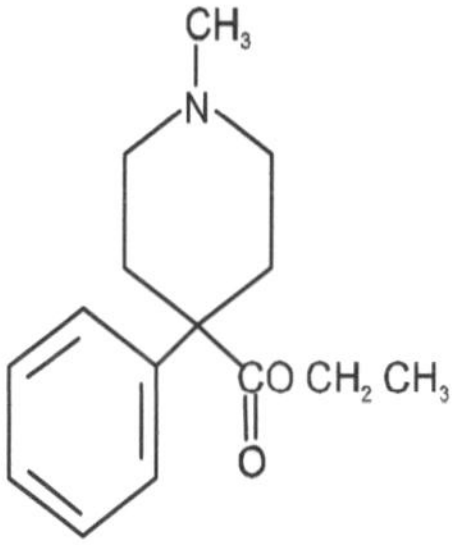

It is synthetic opiods, synthesized as atropine substitute. It interacts with opiod receptor and its action is blocked by naloxone. Its action starts quicker and it is short lasting. It does not suppress cough, miosis, constipation and urinary retention, biliary spasm is less, causes tachycardia, histamine release, sedation, euphoria and local anesthetic action on cornea.

Absorbed both orally and perenterally metabolized in liver and excreted with urine (acidification of urine hastens it).

Therapeutic Uses:

i. Analgesics.
ii. Pre-anesthetic.
iii. To contract shivering from recovery.
iv. Labour.

ADR: Overdose may produce excitation, tremor, hyperreflexia delirium, convulsion (due to accumulation of demethylation product of pethidine that is norpethidine), tolerance, physical dependence.

Cotraindications: Like morphine, raised intracranial pressure, hypersensitivity, dose reduction in hepatic insufficiency (drug is metabolized in liver).

Available as 50,100 mg tab; 100 mg/2 ml inj.

Dose: 50-100 mg I.M. or subcutaneous, I.V. or orally.

TRADE NAME: PETHIDINE HYDROCHLORIDE.

PHENIRAMINE

Enlisted in essential medicine list of India.

This moderately sedative antihistaminic is frequently used antiallergic drug. It is orally and perenterally absorbed, metabolized in liver and excreted with urine, widely distributed including brain.

ADR: Sedation, decreased alertness, light headedness, motor incoordination, dryness of mouth, altered bowel movement, urinary hesitancy, blurred vision, epigastric distress, contact dermatitis on local application. Overdose may produce excitation, hallucination, muscle in- coordination, convulsion, fever and features of belladonna poisoning.

Therapeutic Uses: Allergic disorder, dermatographism, common cold, pruritides.

Available as 25 and 50 mg tab; 15 mg/5 ml syrup, 22.5 mg/ml injections.

TRADE NAME: AVIL.

PHENOBARBITAL

Enlisted both in WHO and Indian essential medicine list.

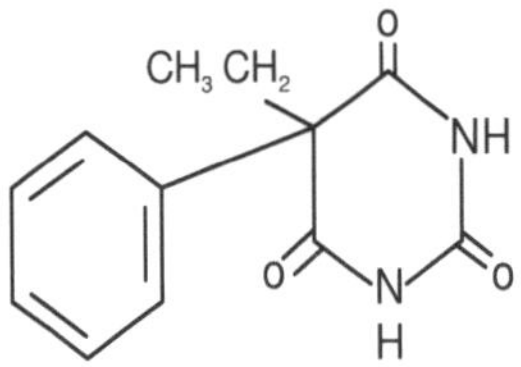

Aside from bromide it in the oldest of the currently available antiseizure drug. It is long acting barbiturates probably the most widely used anticonvulsant.

It is absorbed from G.I.T., widely distributed, penetrates CNS, 20% protein bound, crosses placenta and secreted with milk. Metabolized in liver by oxidation, dealkylation and conjugation.

Therapeutic Uses:

i. Cheapest and least toxic anti-pileptic used for GTC, SP and CP seizures, status epileticus.
ii. Its enzyme inducing property is used for hastening clearance of congenital non-haemolytic jaundice.

ADR: Sedation, rash, megaloblastic anaemia, idiosyncracy (excitement in elderly), tolerance, dependence.

Contraindications: Porphyria, liver and kidney diseases, emphysema, obstructive sleep apnoea.

Interactions:

i. Induces metabolism of warfarin steroid, OCP, tolbutamide, theophylline.
ii. Additive action with alcohol, opioid, antihistaminics.
iii. Sodium valproate increases its level.

Treatment of Phenobarbitone Poisoning

i. Gastric lavage with activated charcol.
ii. Supportive oxygen inhalation, fluid, dopamine, respiratory support.
iii. Alkaline diuresis.
iv. Haemodialysis and haemoperfusion (through column activated charcoal or other absorbent).

Available as 30, 60 mg tab; 20 mg/5 ml syrup. 200 mg/ml injection. TRADE NAME: GARDENAL; PHENOBARBITONE SOD. INJECTION.

PHENYLEPHRINE

Enlisted in Indian essential medicine list.

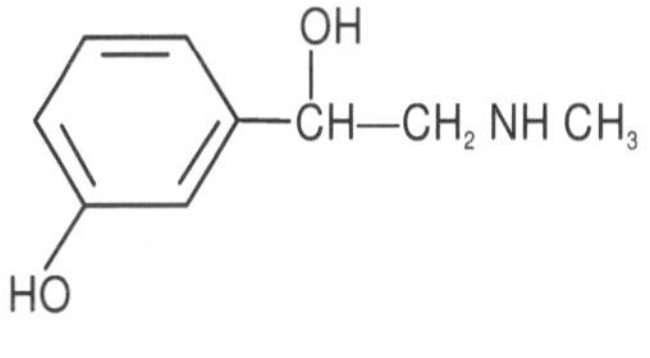

It is widely used topical nasal decongestant. It is selective alpha agonist with negligible β action. It raises BP due to vasoconstriction, there is bradycardia. Other topical uses are mydriasis when cycloplegia is not required.

It reduces intraocular pressure by constricting blood vessels of ciliary body. It is also used orally for nasal decongestant, stronger than 0.25% on topical application on nasal mucosa causes chronic swelling of it.

Dose: 2-5 mg I.M., 01-0.5 mg I.V. slowly 30-60 microgram/min I.V., 5-10 mg oral, 0.25-0.5% nasal instillation; 5-10% eye drops.

Available as 10 mg/ml inj (Frenin). 10% eye drop (Drosin). 0.25% nasal drop (Fenox) with nephazoline 0.025%, 5 mg as tabs with paracetamol etc (Decold).

PHENOXY METHYL PENICILLIN

Included in WHO enlisted essential medicine.

It is acid stable, other properties and spectrum of activities are like penicillin G except it is 1/5 as active against Neisseria. It is orally better absorbed, 25% plasma protein bound, peak plasma level reaches in one hour and plasma t/2 –is ½ - 1 hour. It is not very effective against serious infections.

Therapeutic Uses:

i. Streptococcus pharyngitis.
ii. Sinusitis.
iii. Otitis media.
iv. Prophylaxis to rheumatic fever.
v. Trench mouth.
vi. Less serious pneumococcal infection.

Available as 125, 250 mg tab; 65-130 mg tab; 125 mg/5 ml dry syrup.

Dose: 250-500 mg, infants 60 mg; children 125-250 mg QDS.

TRADE NAME: CRYSTAPEN-V; KAYPEN; PINOVORAL 125 mg of the drug is equivalent to 200,000 units.

PHENYTOIN SODIUM

Enlisted both in WHO and Indian essential medicine list.

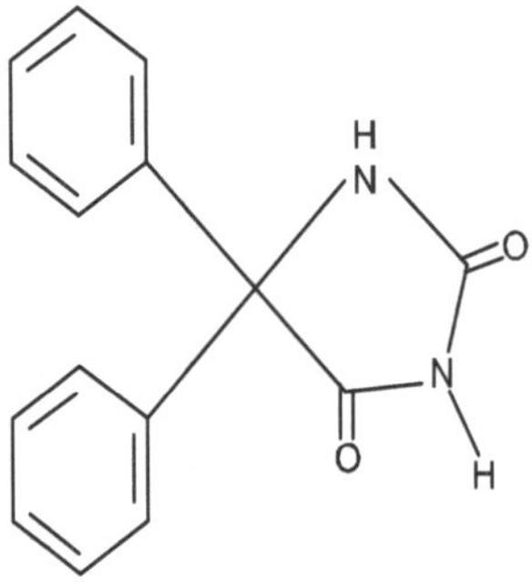

It is perhaps the most useful drug for treating generalized tonic-clonic temporal lobe, or other focal epilepsies and perhaps is the best initial drug chosen particularly in adults. It is often used with phenobarbital or primidone if single agent is not sufficient. It has the advantage of producing little or no sedation in usual doses. It stabilises neuronal membranes of the cells and prevents repetitive detonation during depolarization shift in epileptic patient.

It is slowly absorbed; bioavailability differs in different market preparation, widely distributed, 80-90% protein bound, metabolized in liver by hydroxylation and glucuronide conjugation and kinetics of metabolism shifts from first to zero order.

ADR: Gum hypertrophy, hirsutism; megaloblastic anaemia, osteomalacia; inhibits insulin release; foetal hydantoin syndrome (hypoplastic phalanges, cleft lip; palate, microcephali).

At higher doses: Ataxia, vertigo, diplopia, drowsiness, mental confusion, hallucination, epigastric pain, vomiting, hypotension, arrhythmia.

Available as 25, 50, 100 tab; 100 mg/4 ml/ 5 years; 100 mg/ 2 ml. inj. Fosphenytoin is I.V. preparation; 50 mg/ml in 2 and10 ml container.

TRADE NAME: FOSOLIN.

Dose: 100 mg BD; children 5-8 mg/kg/day.

Therapeutic Uses:

i. Generalized tonic-clonic simple and complex partial seizure.
ii. Status epilepticus.
iii. Trigeminal neuralgia.
iv. Migraine.
v. To reverse digitalis induced arrhythmia.

TRADE NAME : DILANTIN; EPSOLIN.

PHYSOSTIGMINE

Enlisted in Indian essential medicine list.

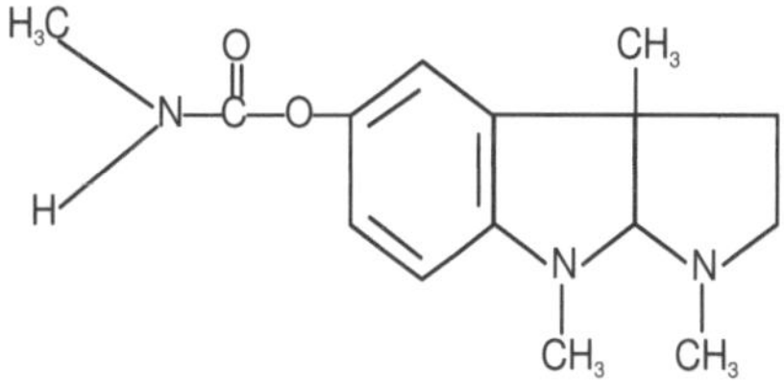

Physostigmine is reversible anticholinesterase chemically carbamates also known as eserine is rapidly absorbed from G.I.T. and perenteral sites, crosses B.B.B.

Therapeutic Uses:

i. Miotic.
ii. Glaucoma.
iii. Belladonna poisoning.
iv. Overdose poisoning to anti-depressant, phenothiazine, antihistaminic.

Available as: Physostigmine salicylate I.P. 0.1 to 1% aqueous solution (on storage it turns pink due to decomposition); 2 mg/ml injection given subcutaneous or I.V. if required every 2-4 hours.

PHYTOMENADIONE

Enlisted in WHO and Indian essential medicine list.

Vitamin K_1 is naphthoquinone derivative lipid soluble vitamin. It is essential for biosynthesis of prothombin that is factor II; proconvertin i.e. VII factor, Christmas factor IX and Stuart Prower factor, i.e., factor X. It probably functions as prosthetic group for an enzyme which is essential for prothombin by hepatic cells. It is also involved in the electron transport (co-enzyme) for oxidative phosphorylation.

Therapeutic Uses:

Hypoprothrombinemia due to:

i. Hepatocellular disease.
ii. Obstructive jaundice.
iii. Newborns.
iv. Oral anticoagulant and salicylate therapies toxicities.

ADR: I.V. use may produce anaphylaxis, haemolytic anaemia, hyperbilirubinemia.

Preparations:

i. Vit K_1 (phytomenadione) 10 mg tab; 10 mg/ml ampoules.
ii. Menadione 5,10 mg tabs; 3 and 10 mg/ml inj.
iii. Menadione sodium bisulfide injection S/C, I.M. or I.V. 1-2 mg daily. In emergencies 10-40 mg I.V. every 4 hours noting prothrombin activitis.
iv. Menadione sodium diphosphate.

TRADE NAME: SYNKAVITE 5 mg tab, 10 mg/ml injection.

PILOCARPINE

Enlisted both in WHO and Indian essential medicine lists.

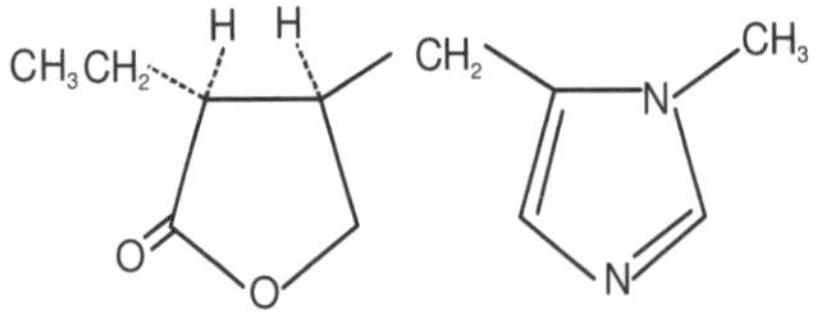

Pilocarpine is an alkaloid obtained from *Pilocarpus microphyllus* and *pilocarpus jaborandi.* It directly stimulates cholinergic innervation (muscarine and nicotine receptors). It stimulates CNS followed by depression.

ADR: G.I. disturbances, salivation, bradycardia, bronchospasm, hypotension, arrhythmia, pulmonary oedema, tingling sensation in eye. It is too toxic for systemic use.

Available is 1, 2 and 4% eye drops.

Therapeutic Uses:

i. Open angle glaucoma.
ii. To counter act mydriatic and to break adhesion of iris from lens.

TRADE NAME: PILOCAR; PILODROPS.

PNEUMOCOCCAL VACCINES

Enlisted in WHO's essential medicine list.

There are two types of pneumococcal vaccines:

i. Pneumococcal polysaccharides conjugated to proteins; and
ii. Bacterial polysaccharides of 23 serotypes both can be given I.M. or S/C. The latter is given as single dose and to repeat every 5 years.

Indications: Adults over 65 years and persons with increased risk of pneumococcal disease or its complications.

PODOPHYLLUM RESINS

WHO enlisted essential medicine.

25% dispersion of podophyllum resin in compound of benzoin tincture or as solution in alcohol is often effective in the treatment of condyloma acuminata, wart, papilloma. It has to be removed after 6 hours of application. Systemic toxicity is reported.

Available as 20% paint (Podowart) 0.5% solution (CONDYLINE).

POLYGELINE

Included in Indian essential medicine list.

This is degraded gelatin polymer, used as plasma expander, polypeptide, average MW 30000 exerts osmotic pressure like albumin. Non antigenic, hypersensitivity is rare but should be watched for it. Does not interfere with blood grouping, cross matching, not metabolized in the body. Expansion for plasma lasts for 12 hours.

ADR: Flushing, rigor, urticaria, wheezing, hypotension.

Therapeutic Uses: Burn, shock (hypovolumic and endotoxic, trauma, tissue damage; temporary measures to blood loss.

Available as 3.5% solution in balanced electrolyte medium in 500 ml container.

Contraindications: Severe anaemia, CCF, pulmonary edema, renal insufficiency.

TRAME NAME: HAEMACCEL; SERACCEL.

POTASSIUM CHLORIDE

WHO and Indian essential medicine enlisted drug.

It is used to treat hypokalemia except in rare condition where there is hyperchloremia.

Therapeutic Uses:

i. Diuretic.
ii. Low K^+ intake.
iii. G.I. loss.
iv. As antidote to digitalis toxicity.
v. Hypokalemic periodic paralysis.
vi. Adjunct to anti cholinesterase drug in myasthenia gravis.
vii. Metabolic alkalosis.

KCL is usually preferred salt, because chloride ion corrects hypokalemia and alkalosis. Most commercial preparations contain 10-40 mEq KCl/15 ml. with flavouring agent to unmask disagreeable taste which is diluted before intake. Uncoated tablets cause gastric irritation I.V. KCl is given if patient can't take it orally and if hypokalemia is severe.

Precaution: Patient receiving potassium sparing diuretics and to renal insufficiency patients.

Available as KCl oral solution; KCl injection.

POTASSIUM IODIDE

WHO enlisted essential medicine.

Therapeutic Uses:

i. Antitussive.
ii. Expectorant.
iii. Hyperthyroidism.
iv. Sporotrichosis.

In all these conditions KI is given orally. For therapy of choice cutaneous lymphatic sporotrichosis 1 mg/ml solution to a patient who can tolerate it. It may produce iodism symptomised by (brassy taste, rhinitis, coryza, salivation, lacrymation, sneezing, burning of mouth and throat, ocular irritation, dermal lesions, sialadenitis), heart burn, nausea and diarrhoea.

POTASSIUM PERMANGANATE

It is included in both WHO and Indian essential medicine list.

These purple crystals are highly soluble in water, liberates oxygen, which oxidizes bacterial protoplasm. The oxygen is germicidal and the solution looses the colour if much organic matter is present. Condy's lotion 1:4000 to 1:10000 is used for gargling, douching, irrigating cavities urethra, wounds. It is also used to disinfect well and ponds, stomach wash for alkaloidal poisoning. It promotes rusting, so not good for sterilizing surgical instruments.

POVIDONE IODINE

Enlisted in WHO and Indian essential medicine list.

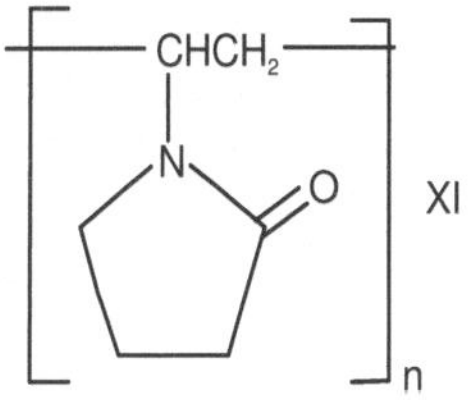

Povidone iodine is an organic iodine—Polyvinylpyrrolidone complex, slowly releasing iodine and the activity of the preparation is directly related to the availability of free iodine.

Therapeutic Uses:

i. Antiseptic to skin, mucous membrane.
ii. To control susceptible cutaneous infection and vaginal in fections.
iii. Infection of mouth, scalp.
iv. Pre operative skin preparation.
v. Trichomonal vaginitis.
vi. Disinfecting endoscopes.

It is less irritating, non-toxic, non-staining, produces prolonged germicidal effects.

Local hypersensitivity may occur.

Available as 5% solution, 5% ointment, 7.5% scrub solution, 1% mouth wash, 200 mg vaginal pessary.

TRADE NAME: BETADINE; PIODINE.

PRALIDOXIME (2-PAM)

Enlisted in Indian essential medicine list.

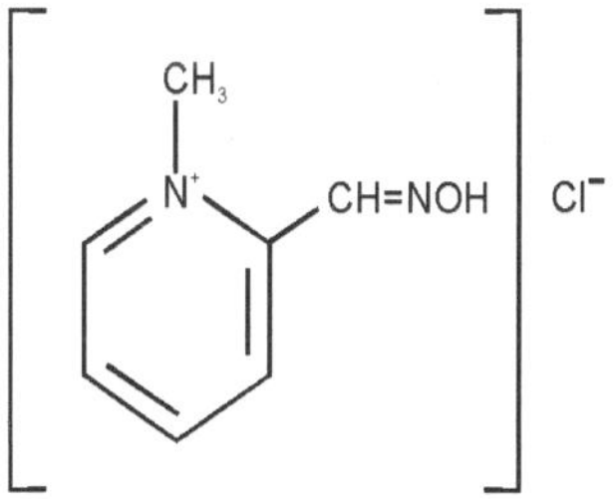

This cholinesterase reactivator is given I.V. as an adjunct to atropine in systemic cholinesterase inhibitor poisoning. Topical administration is ineffective except by sub-conjunctival injection enters the eye in therapeutic concentration. It is occasionally used as a part of drug regimen to break resistant posterior synachea or to obtain maximum mydriasis.

Available as 500 mg/20 ml I.V. infusion.

Dose: 1-2 g I.V. slowly or 20-40 mg/kg slowly. Reactivation of skeletal muscle cholinesterase occurs more markedly and no CNS ChE reactivation because it does not cross BBB.

It is more effective against phosphorylate ChE-I than against carbamylate.

TRADE NAME: NEOPAM; PAM-A.

PRAZIQUANTEL

WHO and Indian essential medicine enlisted drug.

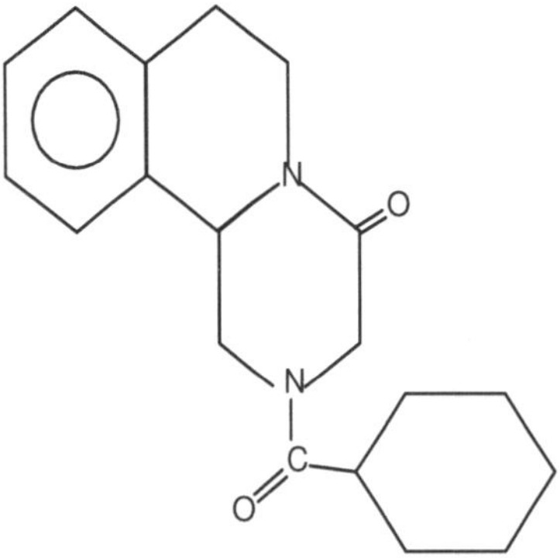

It is synthetic isoquinoline-pyrazine derivative, effective against schistosomes, trematodes, cestodes but not nematodes. It is taken up by susceptible worms and causes contracture paralysis.

Orally absorbed which is hastened by ingesting with food. It has high first pass metabolism. Phenytoin, carbamazepine induce its metabolism. Crosses BBB, metabolites are excreted with urine.

Therapeutic Uses:

i. Tapeworms (H. nana, T. saginata, T. solium, D. latum).
ii. Neurocysticercosis 50-100 mg/kg in three divided doses × 15 days. It is contraindicated in ocular cysticercosis.
iii. Schistosomes 40-75 mg/kg once.
iv. Other flukes except Fasciola hepatica.

Dose: 75 mg/kg/day for 1-2 days.

ADR: Systemic toxicity is less. Bitter taste produces nausea, abdominal pain, headache, sedation, dizziness, itching, urticaria, rash, fever, bodyache.

Does not interact with alcohol, tobacco, food.

Available as 50 mg and 600 mg tabs.

TRADE NAME: CYSTICIDE; DISTOCIDE.

PREDNISOLONE

WHO and Indian essential medicine enlisted drug.

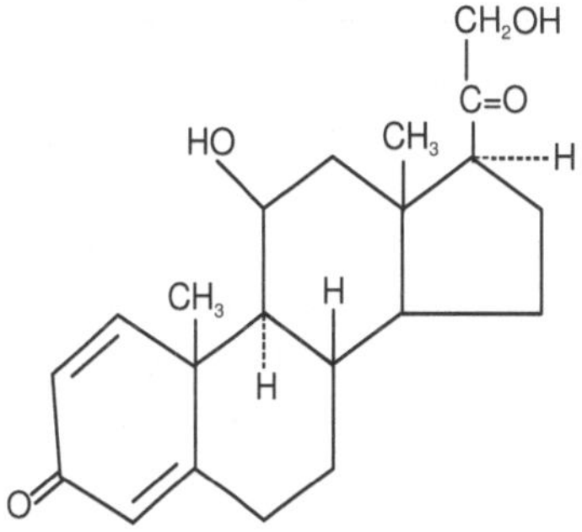

This is synthetic glucocorticoid derivative from hydrocortisone. 5 mg of prednisolone is equivalent to 20 mg of hydrocortisone and with less Na and H_2O retaining property. It is used for the treatment of inflammatory, malignancies and allergic conditions which respond to glucocorticoid but suitable not for adrenocortical insufficiency for which a potent mineralocorticoids such as desoxycortisone or fludrocortisone should be given simultaneously.

Its base is used orally or topically, soluble sodium phosphate or sodium succinate esters can be given I.V. intra-articularly or I.M. tabulate and acetate form may also be used intra-articularly or into soft tissues but these are slowly absorbed or long acting.

Available as 5, 10 mg tab; 20 mg/ml as acetate for I.V. or I.M. and intra-articular injection.

TRADE NAME: DELTACORTRIL; WYSOLONE, NUCORT.

PRIMAQUINE

WHO and Indian essential medicine enlisted drug.

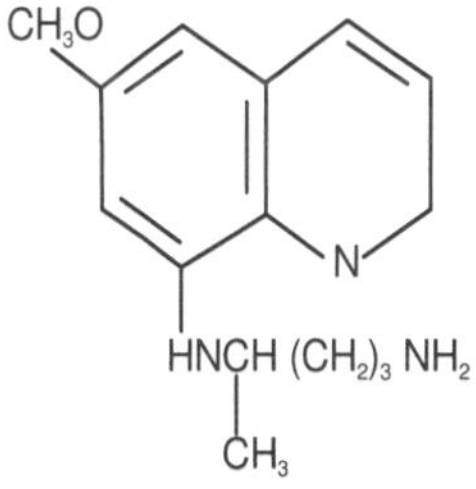

Chemically it is 8-aminoquinoline, causal prophylactic for all species of malaria but not included in mass programme because of its toxicity. The adverse effect is intravascular haemolysis in glucose 6 PO_4 dehydrogenase deficiency. It is also active against gamatocytes.

It is orally absorbed, metabolized in liver and excreted in urine, not cumulative.

ADR: Abdominal pain, G.I. upset, weakness uneasiness can be minimized if taken with food. Other serious toxicity as mentioned earlier haemolysis, methaemoglobinaemia, tachypnoea, cyanosis, should be avoided in pregnancy.

Therapeutic Uses: Radical cure of relapsing P. vivax 15 mg daily (0.25 mg/kg children) for 2 weeks with chloroquine. Alternative regimen 45 mg primaquine and chloroquine 300 mg per week for 8-10 weeks. For P. falciparum: Single 45 mg dose of primaquine with curative dose of chloroquine.

Available as 26 mg as phosphate = 15 mg base 7.5; 15 mg tab.

Other Uses: Pneumocystis jiroveci pneumonia with clindamycin 600 mg + primaquine 15 mg/day.

TRADE NAME: PRIMALINE; MALIRID.

PROCAINAMIDE

WHO and Indian essential medicine enlisted drug.

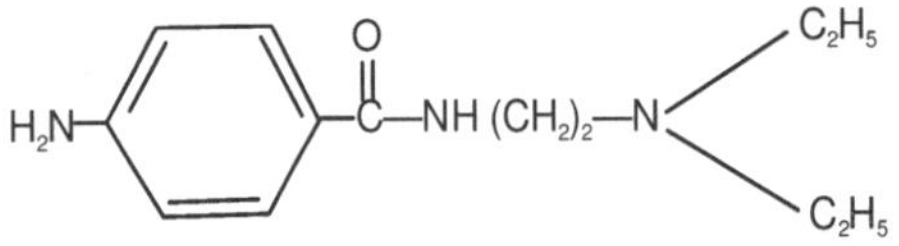

Procainamide belongs to class I antiarrhythmic drug electrophysiologically similar to quinidine of Vaughan William and Singh's (1969) classification of antiarrhythmic drug. It is orally active amide, metabolized in liver by acetylation to N-acetylation procainamide (NAPA) which blocks K^+ channel and prolongs repolarization and APD. There are fast and slow acetylators for its metabolism.

ADR: Nausea, vomiting, weakness, confusion, hallucination, flushing, hypotension, torsade de pointes, fever, rash, agranulocytosis, SLE.

Therapeutic Uses: Monomorphic VT.

Dose: For abolition of arrhythmia 0.5 to 1 gm oral or I.M. followed by 0.25-0.5 g every 2 hours or 500 mg I.V. loading dose (25 mg/min) followed by 2 mg/kg/hour.

Maintenance Dose: 500 mg every (4-6 hours).

Available as 250 mg tab; 1 g/10 ml inj.

TRADE NAME : PRONESTYL.

PROCAINE BENZYL PENICILLIN

WHO and Indian essential medicine enlisted drug.

This is a repository preparation of penicillin. It is available as powder form to be solubilized in distilled water prior to injection.

Dose: 500000-1000000 unit daily I.M. A single I.M. dose peak plasma level reaches after 1-3 hours which is 25 times lower than benzyl penicillin, but it remains in blood for 8-12 hours. Aqueous solution is stable for many months at temperature below 25°C.

Available as 0.5 MU dry powder.

Therapeutic Uses and **ADR** are like benzyl penicillin.

TRADE NAME: PROCAINE PENICILLIN–G.

PROCARBAZINE

Enlisted in WHO and Indian essential medicine list.

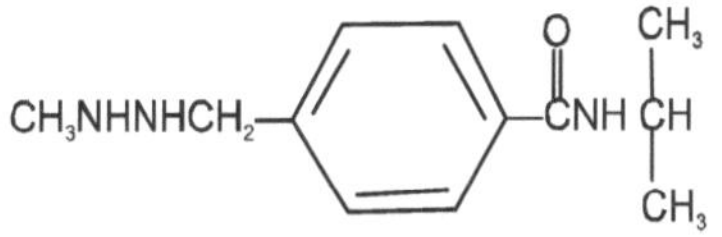

It is synthetic methyl hydrazine derivative.

After metabolic activation, it depolymerizes DNA to cause chromosomal damage. It is popular in MOPP therapy of Hodgkin's disease and other uses are non-Hodgkin's lymphoma and oat cell carcinoma.

ADR: Vomiting, leucopenia, dermatitis, thrombocytopenia.

It has MAO-inhibiting property, so may interact.

Dose: 100 mg/sq mt/day for 14 days in 28 days cycle.

TRADE NAME: INDICARB 20 MG CAP.

PROCHLORPERAZINE

Enlisted in Indian essential medicine list.

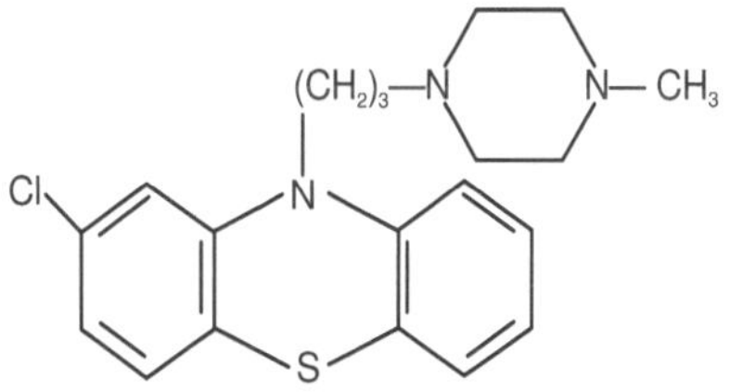

This drug blocks D_2, suppresses labyrinthine and has anti vertigo and antiemetic action.

Therapeutic uses in management of post-operative nausea, vomiting, radiation sickness, nausea and vomiting of toxins. It has significant intrinsically prolong action, so time release preparation has no special advantage.

ADR: Extrapyramidal symptoms, drowsiness, cutaneous reaction, orthostatic hypotension, amenorrhoea, cholestasis, neutropenia, should not be used below 2 years.

Available as Prochlorperazine maleate 5, 25 mg tab; 12.5 mg/ml ampoules, 10 ml vial.

It has also got role in antipsychotic and antimaniac.

TRADE NAME: STEMETIL.

PROGUANIL

WHO enlisted essential medicine.

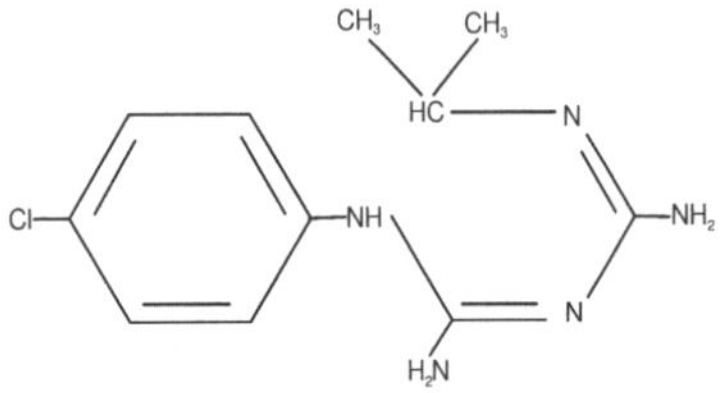

Chemically it is biguanide derivative, slow acting erythrocytic schizontocide, also inhibits pre-erythrocyte stage of P. falciparum. Gametocytes fail to develop when exposed to it. It is cyclized in body to triazines which inhibits plasmodial DHFRase. Resistance occurs due to mutation. Orally absorbed, partly metabolized and excreted with urine.

ADR: Well tolerated, vomiting, stomatitis, haematuria, rash, loss of hair (transient).

Dose: Prophylaxis 200 mg OD+ chloroquine 300 mg weekly × 4 weeks.

It potentiates atovaquione, so used in Thailand as combination.

Available as 100 mg tab.

TRADE NAME: LAVERAN; PROGUNAL.

PROMETHAZINE

Enlisted both in WHO and Indian essential medicine lists.

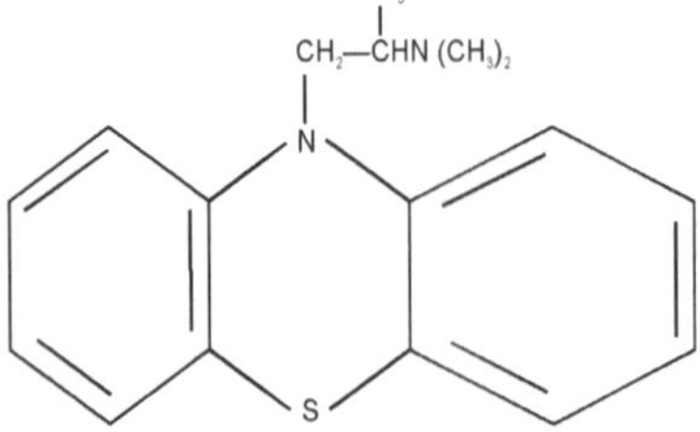

It is less effective in the vomiting caused due to chemoreceptor stimulation. It is effective in motion sickness (labyrinthine suppressant). It has H_1 receptor blocking action. Its sedative helps in the treatment of post operative nausea and vomiting. It is also effective pre-anaesthetic medication (50 mg I.M.) as sedative and anxiolytic. Used as antiparkinsonian due to its central anticholinergic action. Promethazine theoclate commercially available as AVOMINE promoted as antiemetic.

ADR: Drowsiness, orthostatic hypotension. Contraindicated in stuporous, cardiac and cerebrovascular insufficiency patient.

Injections 25 and 50 mg/ml; oral 6.25, 25 mg/5 ml syr; tab 12.5, 25, 50 mg.

Rectal suppositories 25 and 50 mg.

Dose: I.M. oral; rectal 25 mg, and then 12.5 to 25 mg every four to six hours. Children over 3 months of age 0.25 to 0.5 mg/kg four to six times a day.

TRADE NAME: PHENERGAN.

PROPRANOLOL

Enlisted in WHO and Indian essential medicine list.

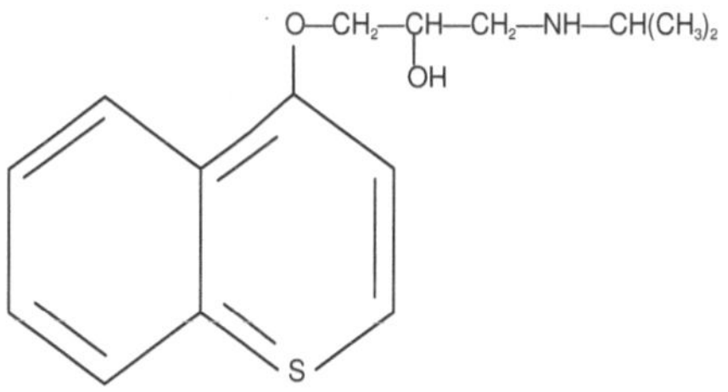

It is non selective β adrenergic antagonist. It is well absorbed orally but bioavailability is low due to high first pass metabolism in the liver. Its metabolism depends upon hepatic blood flow. On prolonged and repeated use its bioavailability increases due to decreased hepatic blood flow. If faken after meal bioavailability increases due to decreased first pass metabolism. Its hydroxylated metabolic product has β blocking property, 90% of it is protein bound.

Dose: Oral 10-160 mg QDS, average 40-60 mg/day I.V. 2-5 mg over 10 minutes with monitoring. It is not given I.V. or s/c because it is irritant.

Available as 10, 40, 80 mg tab 1 mg/ml injection.

Therapeutic Uses: Hypertension, sinus tachycardia, AF, antianginal, portal hypertension, migraine, thyrotoxicosis, intention tremor, anti anxiety.

ADR: Myocardial insufficiency, bradycardia, prinzmetal's angina, carbohydrate intolerance, raises LDL cholesterol, withdrawl should be gradual. Bronchial asthma, heart block, worsening peripheral vascular diseases, nightmare, forgetfulness, sexual distress, hallucination, reducing exercise capacity due to decrease of muscle blood flow.

TRADE NAME: INDERAL; CIPLAR.

PROPYLTHIOURACIL

WHO enlisted essential medicine.

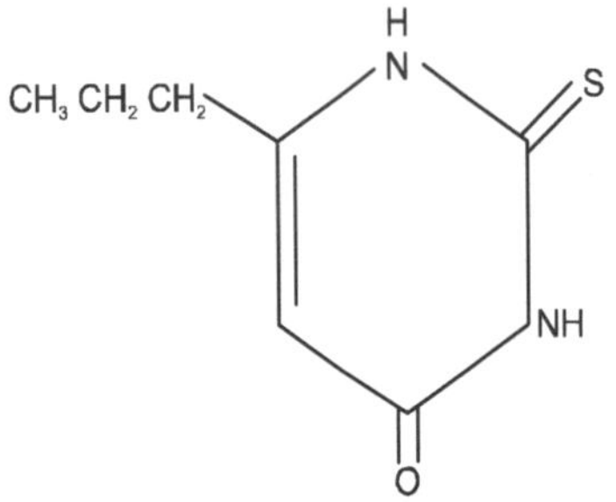

This is the prototype of antithyroid drug used for management of hyperthyroidism, preoperative preparation of thyroidectomy patient, thyrotoxic crisis, also given before or after radioactive iodine.

ADR: Agranulocytosis (requires withdrawl), pruritis, rash, nausea, arthralgia, abdominal discomfort, headache, dizziness, paresthesia, loss of taste, drug fever, hepatitis, nephritis, alopecia, depigmentation of hair, recurrent keratitis, resembling connective tissue disorder may be given to pregnant women with small dose 200-300 mg in first half and 100-150 mg in later half, it crosses placental barrier.

It is orally absorbed, widely distributed in the body, crosses placenta, enter milk, metabolized in liver and excreted with urine.

Dose: 50-150 mg tab followed by 25-50 mg tab BD to TDS as maintenance.

Available as 50 mg tab.

TRADE NAME: PTU.

PROTAMINE SULFATE

Enlisted both in WHO and Indian essential medicine list

This low molecular protein is strongly basic compound, source is sperms of some fishes given I.V. to neutralize the effect of heparin (1mg of protamine sulfate neutralizes 100 I.V. of heparin). Generally used when heparin's action to be terminated quickly (as for example after cardiac and valvular surgery).

In absence of heparin it acts as anticoagulant by interacting with platelets and fibrinogen.

ADR: Releases histamine, hypersensitivity, flushing, breathing difficulty.

Available as 50 mg/5 ml injection.

TRADE NAME: PROTA; PROTAMINE SULFATE.

PRUSSIAN BLUE

WHO enlisted essential medicine.

It is very dark blue, color fast, non toxic, pigment discovered in Berlin. It is inorganic compound with idealized formula$(Fe)_7 (CN)_{18}$, containing also variable amounts of water and other ions. Despite presence of cyanide ions, it is not poison because it is tightly bound.

Used as antidote of heavy metal poisoning (thallium or radioactive cesium). An adult male can eat at least 10 gm of Prussian blue without any serious harm.

Available as 500 mg prussian blue capsules.

It is a common stain used by pathologist to detect presence of iron in biopsy specimen of bone marrow.

PYRANTEL PAMOATE

Enlisted both in WHO and Indian essential medicine list.

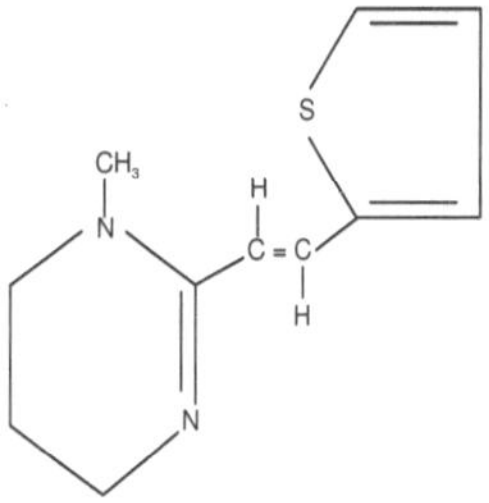

This is highly effective in thread worm, round worm, hook worm and given as a single dose.

It causes persistent depolarization of the worm resulting from nicotinic cholinergic receptor leading to contracture and spastic paralysis.

ADR: Anorexia, nausea, vomiting, diarrhoea, abdominal pain, headache, dizziness, drowsiness, rash, SGOT is raised.

Dose: 10 mg/kg, 3 days course recommended for necator and strongyloides. No preparation is required. May be repeated after 1 month.

Available as 250 mg tab, 50 mg/ml in 10 ml/bottle.

TRADE NAME: NEMOCID; ANTIMINTH.

PYRAZINAMIDE

Enlisted both in WHO and Indian essential medicine list.

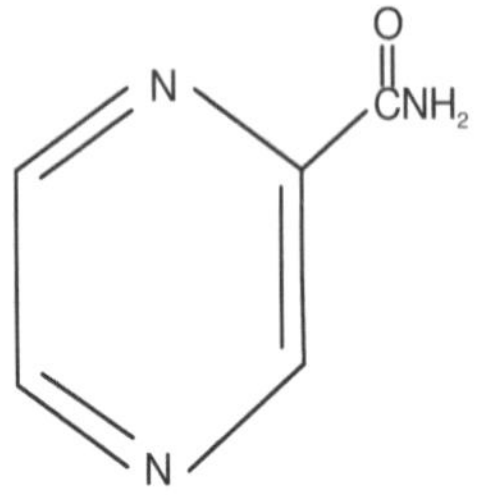

This analogue of nicotinamide is insoluble in water. Most physicians use it for retreatment because of its potential toxicity. It is more active in acidic media more lethal to intracellularly located bacteria. Highly effective in first 2 months. It inhibits mycolic acid synthesis.

It is orally absorbed, widely distributed with good CSF penetration, metabolized in liver and excreted with urine.

ADR: Hepatotoxicity, arthralgia, flushing fever, hyperuricaemia, loss of diabetes control.

Available as 0.5; 0.75; 1 g tab; 250 mg/5 ml syrup.

Dose: 25-30 mg/kg/day.

TRADE NAME: PYZINA; PZA-CIBA.

PYRIDOSTIGMINE

Enlisted both in WHO and Indian essential medicine list.

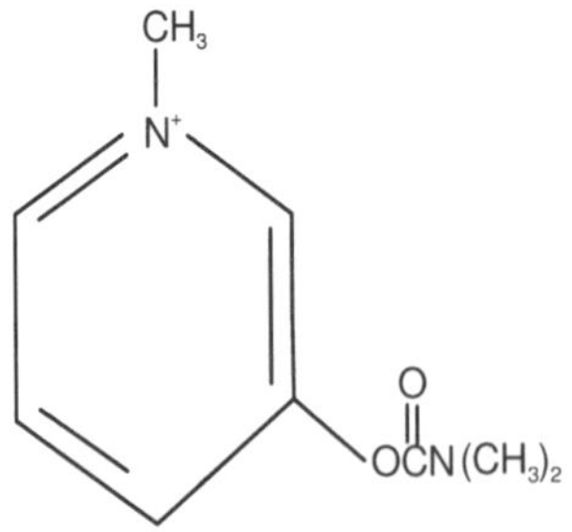

It is given orally to treat myasthenia gravis. It is carbamate derivative acts as reversible anti-cholinesterase. It resembles neostigmine in all aspect, except dose to dose less potent and longer acting.

Available as 60 mg tabs of pyridostigmine bromide.

Dose: 1-3 tabs TDS.

ADR: Rarely/produce ADR in therapeutic doses. Higher dose may cause cholinergic crisis. Patient sensitive to bromide may cause skin reactions. Use with caution in bronchial asthma patients.

PYRIDOXINE

Enlisted both in WHO and Indian essential medicine list.

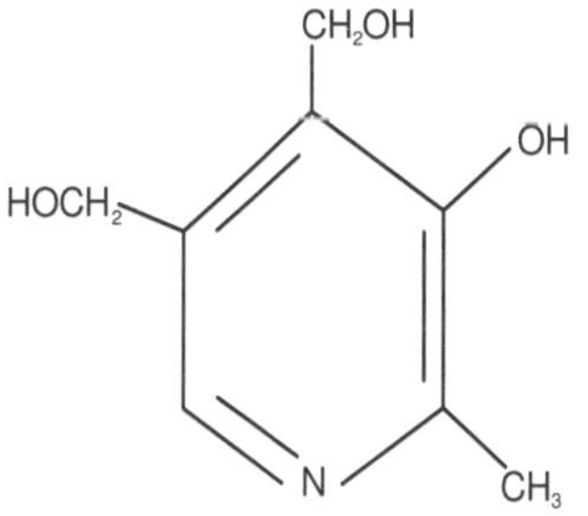

This is one of component of B_6 vitamin (others are pyridoxal, pyridoxamine) which are all functionally and metabolically interrelated.

Found in whole grains, cereals, peanuts, corn.

Therapeutic Uses

i. Infants with epileptiform convulsions.
ii. Hypochromic anaemia.
iii. Homocystinuria.
iv. Peripheral neuritis.
v. With INH, hydralazine, penicillamine.
vi. After peritoneal dialysis.
vii. Nausea and vomiting in pregnancy.
viii. To reverse increased level of tryptophan metabolism that occur in some patient taking OCP.

Do not give to patient taking levodopa.

Available as 10, 25, 50, 100 tabs; 50 mg/ml in 10 ml container.

Dose: Oral 5-10 mg OD, Inj. 25-100 mg I.M. or I.V.

PYRIMETHAMINE + SULFADOXINE

WHO and Indian essential medicine enlisted drug.

This fixed drug combination is approved for P. falciparum. Pyrimethamine is directly acting inhibitor of plasmodial DHFRase.

Available as Sulfadoxin 500 mg + Pyrimethamine 25 mg.

Dose: For clinical curative: Sulfadoxine 1500 mg + pyrimethamine 75 mg single dose (3 tabs). Children 9-14 years 2 tabs. Children 4-8 years 1 tab. Children 1-4 years ½ tab.

TRADE NAME: LARIDOX; REZIZ.

QUINIDINE

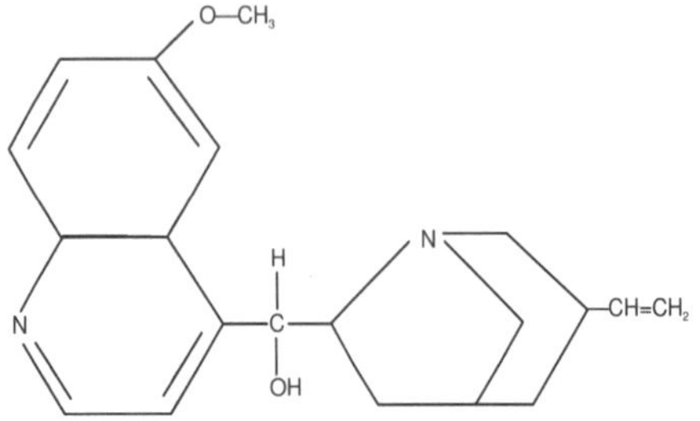

It is class IA antiarrhythmic agent. Moderately decreases dv/dt of phase O. It is dextrose-isomer of alkaloid quinine obtained from cincona bark. It increases, PR,Q-T interval and broadens QRS complex. Available as 200 mg tab, 600 mg/2 ml injection.

Therapeutic Uses: Atrial flutter or fibrillation or maintain sinus rhythm after terminating them.

Dose: 100-200 mg TDS.

Angioedema, vascular collapse,thrombocytopenia may occur as ADR.

QUININE

Enlisted in WHO and Indian essential medicine list.

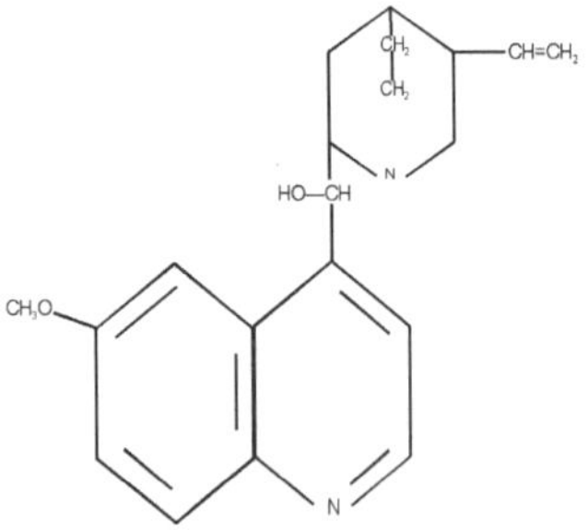

It is levo-rotatory alkaloid of cinchona bark. It is erythrocytic schizontocides for all species of malaria, also respond to most chloroquine and multi drug resistant *P. falciparum.*

It is orally absorbed, 70% plasma proteins (α_1 acid glycoprotein). Metabolized in liver by CYP3A4 and excreted in urine. It is cumulative.

Its toxicity is high. Large high dose produces cinchonism manifest as nausea, ringing in ear, confusion, vertigo, visual defects, diarrhoea, flushing, perspiration which all subsides on stopping the drugs.

Poisoning manifest as tachypnoea, respiratory depression, weakness, fever, prostration, hypotension, cardiac arrhythmia.

Occasionally haemolysis, black water fever, kidney damage. It should be avoided in pregnancy. Hypoglycemia may occur.

Available as 300 mg, 600 mg tab; 600 mg/2 ml inj. Other actions are local irritants and anesthetics, abortificients, analgesic, antipyretic.

Therapeutic Uses

i. Malaria: Uncomplicated: 600 mg TDS for 3-7days.
   Complicated: Cerebral malaria (10 mg/kg/I.V. over 1-2 hours then 0.02 mg/kg/I.V.) per minute.
ii. Nocturnal muscle cramps 200-300 mg at bed time.
iii. In diagnosis of myasthenia gravis.
iv. In varicose vein it is injected with urathane which causes thrombosis → fibrosis → obliteration of varicose vein.
v. Myotonia congenita.

RABIES IMMUNOGLOBULIN

It is included in WHO and Indian essential medicine list.

It is also called "equine rabies immunoglobulin". It is refined, concentrated and lyophilized serum from horse by repeated injection of fixed rabies virus. It is given simultaneously with rabies vaccine 40 I.U. is infiltrated around the wound and rest is injected I.M.

Available as 1000 I.U./5 ml inj.

It is inferior to rabies immunoglobulin human (HRIG).

TRADE NAME: IMORAB.

RABIES VACCINE

Included in WHO and Indian essential medicine list.

Four types of rabies vaccines are available.

i. **Antirabies vaccine carbolized (sample vaccine):** Also called neural tissue vaccine (NTV). Given 14 daily (2-5 ml) of injections in anterior abdominal wall. Obsolete now.
ii. **Purified chick embryo cell vaccine (PCEV):** Marketed as Rabipur. Given 1ml over deltoid muscle. It is Flury-LEP strain of rabies virus grown in chick fibroblast and inactivated by betapropiolactone 2.5 I.U./ml.
   Local pain, erythema, swelling of lymph node and rarely neuroparalytic complications may arise.
iii. **Human diploid cell vaccine (HDCV):** Rabies virus grown in human diploid cell culture, inactivated and lyophilized 2.5 I.U./ml (freshly prepared with diluent).
   Redness induration rarely encephalitis may occur.

iv. **Purified vero cell rabies vaccine (PVRV):** It contains inactivated wister rabies PM/W 138-1-503-3M strain grown in vero continuous cell line. Marketed as verorab 1 ml.

RALOXIFENE

Included in essential medicine list of India.

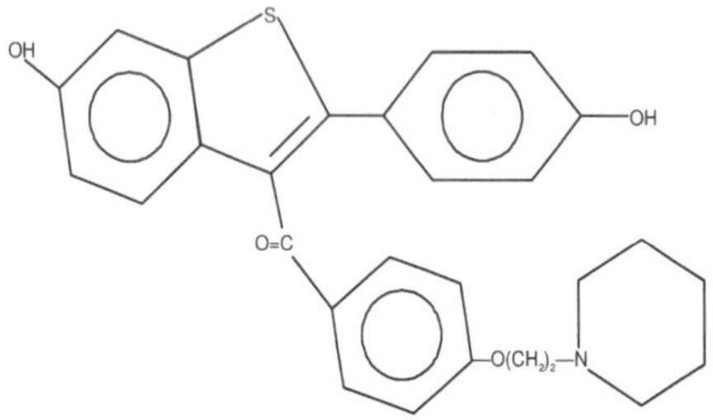

Raloxifene is selective oestrogen receptor modulator with partial agonist action on bone and CVS but antagonist to endometrium and breasts. It has distinct DNA target. Raloxifene response element REE. It increases bone mass, decrease LDL cholesterol in post menopausal women. Orally absorbed, high first pass effect by glucuronidation decreases bioavailability, excreted with faeces.

Side Effects: Leg cramps, hot flushes, vaginal bleeding, deep vein thrombosis and pulmonary embolism.

Used for osteoporosis in female in post menopausal woman.

Dose: 60 mg/day.

Available as 60 mg tab.

TRADE NAME: BONMAX; RALOTAB.

RANITIDINE

Enlisted in Indian essential medicine list.

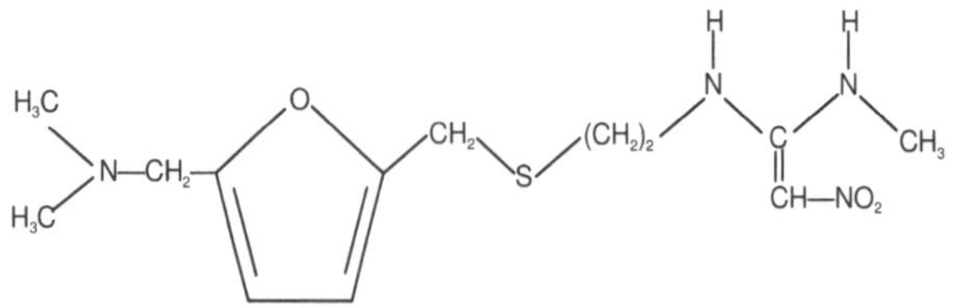

This is H_2 receptor for blocker. Therapeutically used for (i) Duodenal ulcer (ii) Gastric ulcer (iii) Stress ulcer and gastritis (iv) Zollinger-Ellison syndrome (v) Gastro esophageal reflux disease (vi) In association with NSAID and steroids (ulcerogenic drug) (vii) Prophylaxis to aspiration pneumonia (viii) In certain urticaria with H_1 blocker.

Given orally; IM or IV.

Dose: 150 mg BD or 300 mg at bed time. For gastrinoma 300 mg 3-4 times/day.

Perenteral dose 50 mg IM or slowly IV every 6-8 hours. Rapid IV administration may cause hypotension, 0.1- 0.25 mg/kg/hour IV for stress ulcer.

Available as 150 and 300 mg tab; 50 mg/2 ml injection.

Advantages over Cimetidine

i. More potent long acting.
ii. No antiandrogenic effect.
iii. Lesser brain penetration.
iv. Hepatic metabolism is less inhibited.

TRADE NAME: RANTAC; ZINETAC.

RESERPINE

Included in WHO's essential medicine list.

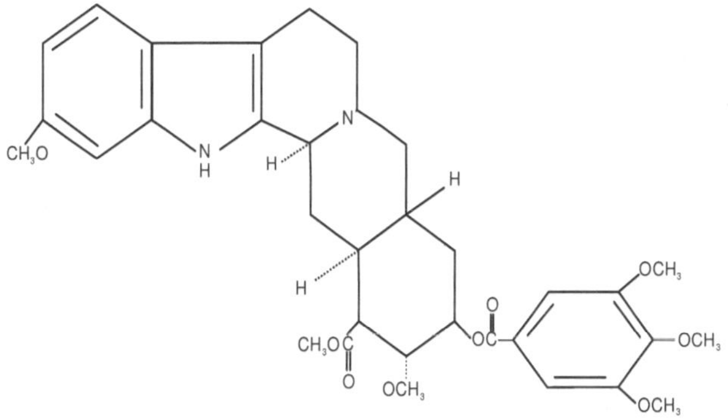

Reserpine is obtained from *Rauwolfia serpentina* a climbing shrub indigenous to India.

The active principal reserpine causes depletion of catecholamine and 5HT. It is used therapeutically as (i) Antipsychotic (ii) Antihypertensive (iii) Tardine dyskinesia (iv) Raynaud's disease and other peripheral vascular diseases associated with increase sympathetic activity.

It can be given orally or I.M. It is taken up by lipid rich tissues and distributed uniformly in various parts of CNS. So may produce cumulative toxicity.

ADR: Salivation, nasal congestion, increased gastric secretion and gut motility, orthostatic hypotension, weight gain, mental depression, parkinsonism, gynaecomastia, impotence, thrombocytopenia and purpura.

Available as:

i. Rauwolfia tabs 4 mg of alkaloids dose 2-4 mg.

ii. Reserpine tab 0.25 mg of reserpine 0.25 to 1 mg daily.
iii. Reserpine injection.

Available as 2 and 10 ml ampoules 2.5 mg/ml given I.M. or I.V. TRADE NAME: SERPASIL.

RETINOL (VITAMIN A)

It is included in WHO and Indian essential medicine list. Discussed with concentrated Vit A solution.

RIBOFLAVIN (VITAMIN B_2)

Included in WHO and Indian essential medicine list.

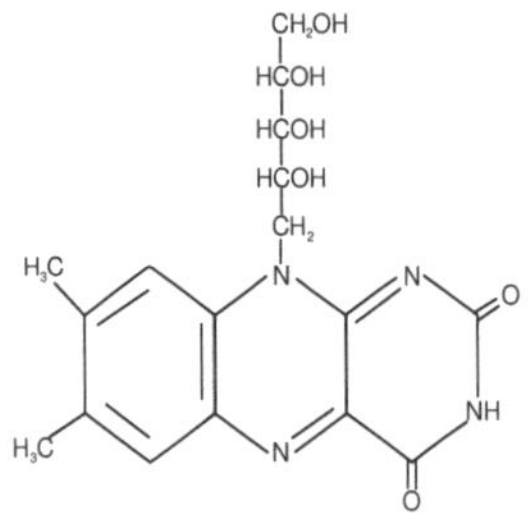

It acts as a co-enzyme playing vital role in the metabolism of respiratory proteins and biological oxidations and maintains RBC's integrity. It is obtained from milk, egg, meat, nuts, green vegetables. Daily requirement 2 mg. Ariboflavinosis is characterised by glositis, angular stomatitis, cheilosis, seborrheic, dermatitis, corneal vascularization. Its deficiency seldom occurs alone. Generally observed with other B. complex deficiency.

It is well absorbed by active transport and phosphorylated in intestine. Body does not store it significantly.

Available as tab 20 g (LIPABOL).

Injections 10 mg/ml (Riboflavin).

No toxic effect of riboflavin is reported in man.

RIFAMPICIN

Included in WHO and Indian essential medicine list.

Rifampicin is semisynthetic derivative of Rifamycin-B obtained from *S. mediterranei.* It inhibits DNA dependent RNA synthesis. Effective against M.tuberculosis, *M.leprae*, *S.aureus*, *N. meningitidis*, *H.influenzae, E. coli, klebsiella*, Pseudomonas, Proteus, Legionella.

Resistance occurs due to mutation of repo B gene. It is orally absorbed, widely distributed, penetrates cavities, caseous mass, placenta and meninges. It is metabolized in liver to deacetylated metabolite, undergoes enterohepatic circulation and excreted with bile and urine.

ADR: Hepatitis, respiratory syndromes (breathlessness, shock, collapse); cutaneous syndromes (flushing pruritis, redness of eyes); flu like syndrome and abdominal syndrome (nausea, vomiting, pain abdomen). Urine and other secretion turns orange red but it is harmless (patient should be told about this).

Interactions: It induces hepatic enzymes so enhances metabolism of many drugs like warfarin; OCP, sulfonylurea, digoxin, steroids.

Available as 150, 300, 600 mg caps; 100/5 ml syr.

To be taken in empty stomach 1 hour before or 2 hours later of meals.

Other Therapeutic Uses:

i. Leprosy.
ii. MRSA diphtheroids and legionella.
iii. Brucellosis with doxycycline.
iv. Prophylaxis to *H.influenza* and meningococcal meningitis.

TRADE NAME: R.CIN ZUCOX.

RINGER-LACTATE SOLUTION

It is included in Indian essential medicine list.

It is indicated like normal saline. Like diarrhea, to stable effective extracellular fluid volume and circulation after surgery with normal kidney function and to postpone the need of blood transfusion temporarily by maintaining plasma volume. It contains:

Na^+	130 mEq	per 1000 ml
K^+	4 mEq	
Ca^{2+}	3 mEq	
Cl^-	109 mEq	
Lactate	28 mEq	

RITONAVIR

Included in WHO and Indian essential medicine list.

Ritonavir is protease inhibitor effective against HIV -1 and 2.

Orally absorbed: High bioavailability.

Available as 600 mg tab.

Dose: 600 mg BD.

It inhibits CYP3A4 enzyme, so susceptible to drug interaction.

ADR: Nausea, diarrhea, paraesthesia may occur.

TRADE NAME: RITOVIR 250 mg tab.

ROXITHROMYCIN

It is included in Indian essential medicine list.

This is long acting, semisynthetic, acid stable antibiotic of macrolide group.

Activity: *Branh catarrhalis, Gard Vaginalis, Legionella.* It is orally absorbed, with better tissue penetration. Less drug interactions than erythromycin because of less affinity for cytochrome P450. (Don't use with cisapride and terfenadine).

Used for R.T.I., ENT, skin and soft tissue infection.

Available as 50 mg, 150 mg, 300 mg tab 50 mg/5 ml 5 syr.

Dose: 150-300 mg BD. Children 2.5-5 mg/kg BD.

TRADE NAMES: ROXID; RULIDE.

RUBELLA VACCINES

Include in WHO essential medicine list.

It contains live attenuated rubella virus (Wistar RA 27/3 strain 1000 $TCID_{50}$ per 0.5 ml injection). Given 0.5 ml IM or deep S/C in upper limb.

Used generally in girls 1 year to puberty. It is generally combined with measles and mumps vaccine (MMR). It protects against German measles. Don't give to pregnant woman, TB patient and in febrile condition.

ADR: Fever, malaise, sore throat, joint pain, lymphadenopathy.

TRADE NAME: R-VAC.

SALBUTAMOL

Enlisted in WHO and Indian essential medicine list.

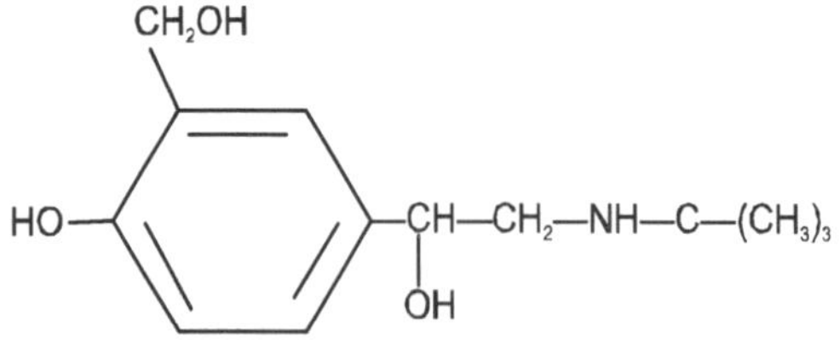

Salbutamol is highly selective β_2 agonist with minimal cardiac side effects. It acts on β_2 receptor to produce increased cAMP formation which sequester Ca^{2+} within sarcoplasmic reticulum to relax the bronchial smooth muscles. It becomes more bronchial specific if given by inhalation and by this route it produces bronchodilation within 5 minutes and it lasts for 2-4 hours.

ADR: Palpitation, nervousness, throat irritation, ankle oedema, palpitation may occur.

Dose: 2-4 mg orally (reserved for those who can't correctly use inhaler). Oral salbutamol is 50% bioavailable and action lasts for 4-6 hours. 0.25-0.5 mg IM or S/C; 100-200 microgram by inhalation.

Available as 2,4 mg tab, 8 mg SR tab.

2 mg/5 ml syrup, 100 microgram/metered dose inhaler, 0.5 mg/ml injection.

TRADE NAME: ASTHALIN; VENTORLIN; CROYSAL as injection.

SALICYLIC ACID

Enlisted in WHO and Indian essential medicine list.

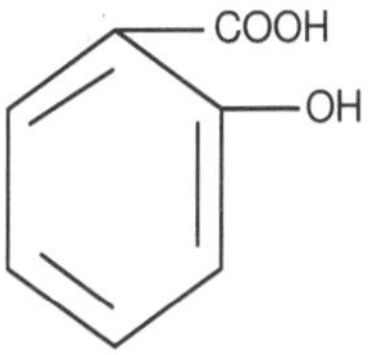

When applied in ointment base in concentration of 3-6%. It is keratolytic, above this concentration it is destructive and below 3% it is keratogenic more than 40% concentration as plaster is used to treat corn and warts, and 10-20% salicylic acid in collodion is used for the same purpose.

Therapeutic Uses: Superficial fungal infection, seborrheic dermatitis, acne, psoriasis, localized neurodermatitis.

It is absorbed even from small lesion to produce salicylism.

SAQUINAVIR

Included in WHO and Indian essential medicine list.

It is protease inhibitors, used for HIV infection. Its original formulation was hard gel capsule was poorly bioavailable, so replaced by soft gel capsule for better bioavailability. It is combined with ritonavir which decreases the gastrointestinal side effects.

Mutation causes resistance. It poorly enters CSF, excreted with faeces.

ADR: Nausea, diarrhea, abdominal discomfort, rhinitis, dyspepsia. It is weak inhibitor of CYP3A4.

Dose: 1200 mg TDS in full stomach and 1000 mg BD if taken with 100 mg of ritonavir.

Available as 200 mg tab.

TRADE NAME: SAQUIN.

SELENIUM SULFIDE

It is enlisted in WHO's and essential medicine list.

It is a drug when applied to the scalp as 2.5% lotion or shampoo, acts as anti-seborrheics (i.e. drug effective for seborrheic dermatitis). Yeast *Pityrosporium ovale* has role in its genesis.

i. Selenium sulfide slows epidermal slowing and scaling.
ii. Antikeratolytic.
iii. Fungicidal to *P. ovale.*

It also helps in dryness and folliculitis.

ADR:

i. Relapse on discontinuation.
ii. Sensitivity.
iii. Toxicity from systemic absorption if applied to denuded skin.

Available as 2.5% suspension.

TRADE NAME: SELSUN.

SENNA

Included in WHO's essential medicine list.

Senna is anthraquinone derivative; irritant purgative obtained from leaves and pods of *Cassia* species, while cascara sagrada is the powdered burk of the buck thorn tree. It passes to colon, where bacteria liberate the active form, which either act locally or absorbed into circulation and excreted via bile to act on small intestine. Bowel is evacuated after 6-8 hours. It is excreted with milk and may cause purging in infants if taken by lactating mother.

ADR: Cramps, excessive purging, inhibit salt and water absorption from colon. PGE2 is also involved in its action (Action blocked by NSAID), rash, fixed drug reaction, regular use may cause colonic atony and mucosal pigmentation.

Available as sennosides as calcium salt 11.5 mg tab.

TRADE NAME: GLAXENNA.

SILVER NITRATE

Enlisted in Indian essential medicine list.

It is available as colourless or white crystals, soluble in water. It is antiseptic, astringent and caustic 1% aquous solution is used as eye drop for conjuntivitis and ophthalmia neonatorum and in treatment of burn. Silver nitrate stick is used to remove warts and small growth of skin and cauterization of trachoma follicle.

ADR: If ingested, produce G.I. tract irritation, vertigo, coma and convulsion.

SILVER SULFADIAZINE

Included in WHO and Indian essential medicine list.

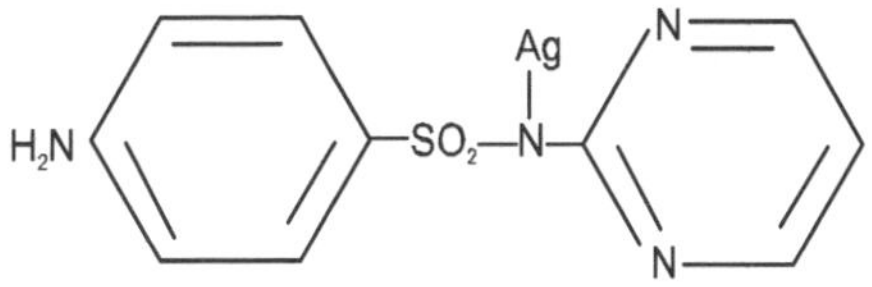

Silver sulfadiazine is used to treat 2nd and 3rd degree burn locally in which it is more active to common gram positive and gram negative organism and reduce mortality. Its spectrum includes *Pseudomonas, Enterobacter,* Klebsiella, *E.coli, Proteus, Staph. strepto, Candida* and *Herpes* virus. It prevents partial thick burn to full thickness burn. Epithelialization can take place in 10 days in favourable condition.

ADR: Pruritis, rash, burning sensation, prolong administration can produce systemic toxicity.

Available as 1% cream.

TRADE NAME: SILVIRIN.

SIMVASTATIN

Included in WHO's essential medicine list.

This stain is used to treat hyperlipidaemic condition, more potent than lovastatin. Increases HDL cholesterol. It is given in lactone precursor form. Orally absorbed, first pass metabolism is extensive.

Dose: 5-20 mg/day.

Available as 5, 10, 20 mg tab.

TRADE NAME: ZOSTA; SIMCARD.

SODIUM CALCIUM EDETATE

Included in WHO's and Indian essential medicine list.

This chelating agent chelates Pb, Zn, Cd, Mn, Cu and some radioactive metals and can remove them from body by exchanging with calcium held by it. Since it is highly ionized so distributed extracellularly. It has to be given I.V. It is excreted by glomerular filtration and excretion.

ADR: Thrombophlebitis, nausea, diarrhea, nephrosis, oliguria, ARF (reversible following drug withdrawl), fever, myalgia, rhinorrhoea, dermatitis, lacrymation).

Preparation: Sodium calcium edetate 20% W/V. It is diluted with normal saline or 5% dextrose.

Available as 20 ml ampoules containing 3 gm of drug in aqueous solution.

Dose: For Pb poisoning 40 mg/kg BD as 0.5 to 3% solution in normal saline or 5% dextrose for 2-3 days. Dose should be less for encephalopathy and in raised intracranial pressure.

It is also used for porphyria, Fe, cadmium, plutonium toxicity.

SODIUM CHLORIDE

Included in WHO's essential medicine list.

It is used for NaCl:

i. As emetic in poisoning.
ii. Mucolytic: Isotonic, NaCl is inhaled by nebulizer helps in the liquification and expectoration of viscid sputum. Evaporated aerosol of NaCl is hypertonic and it is effective in cystic fibrosis. Available as 0.5 m sodium chloride in generic name in USA for nebulizer.
iii. Hypertonic NaCl 3% is used to remove cerumen by irrigating external ear; if tympanic membrane is intact.
iv. Combined therapy of saline with loop diuretic is used for hypercalcemia patient.
v. In metabolic alkalosis it is infused to provide chloride ions.
vi. As O.R.S. and perenteral therapy. Hypertonic NaCl is given for severe hyponatremic patient.

Precaution of NaCl Infusion:

i. CCF.
ii. Circulatory insufficiency, Renal failure, Hypoproteinemia, Hypertonic NaCl should be given slowly in small volumes.

ADR: Pulmonary and peripheral edema.

SODIUM FLUORIDE

It is enlisted in WHO's essential medicine list.

Fluoride is essential through out life, the optimum concentration of 0.7 to 1.2 ppm should be present in drinking water, which reduces the incidence of caries. Caries can also be prevented by applying topical gel of NaF to the tooth.

Chronic fluoride toxicity causes fluorosis occurs due to accidental ingestion of fluoride containing insecticides or inhalation of industrial dust.

Available as:

i. Tabs 1.1, 2.2 mg.
ii. Oral solutions 0.44, 1.1, 3.3, 5.5 and 6.6 mg/ml.
iii. Topical gel drops 11 mg/ml in 24 ml container.

Dose: 1 mg of fluoride, i.e., 2.2 mg of NaF.

SODIUM HYDROGEN CARBONATE

Enlisted in WHO and Indian essential medicine list.

Therapeutically used for:

i. Antiperspirants (applied topically).
ii. For gastric discomfort (as antacid if patient does not require long term treatment and sodium restriction is not required).
iii. In hyperkalemia: 7.5% of $NaHCO_3$ infused to reduce hyperkalemia which shifts potassium into cells.
iv. In hypotensive state: The metabolic acidosis due to hypotension causing accumulation of acid metabolite is treated by infusing $NaHCO_3$ cautiously.
v. In metabolic acidosis.
vi. In peptic ulcer.

SODIUM LACTATE

Included in WHO's essential medicine list.

It is metabolized to sodium bicarbonate in liver and is used to treat metabolic acidosis.

Contains 167 mg/L of Na^+ and lactate 167 mg E/L.

SODIUM NITRITE

Enlisted in WHO and Indian essential medicine list.

It is used to treat cyanide poisoning.10 ml of 3% solution of sodium nitrite is infused intravenously to treat cyanide poisoning which has high affinity for cyanide radical and forms cyanomethaemoglobin. 50 ml of 25% solution of sodium thiosulfate given simultaneously to excrete it out as sodium thiocyanate.

SODIUM NITROPRUSSIDE

Included both in WHO and Indian essential medicine list.

Therapeutic Uses:

i. As antihypertensive.
ii. In CCF.
iii. In myocardial infarction.
iv. As adjunct to anesthesia.
v. In peripheral vascular disorders.

It is quick and consistently acting vasodilator with brief duration of action (2-5 min). It decreases vascular resistance → venous return is reduced → Cardiac output is reduced.

The endothelial cells and RBC splits Na-nitroprusside to generate NO, which relaxes the vascular smooth muscles. It is non-enzymatically converted to NO and CN by glutathione.

Doses: Hypertensive emergencies, 50 mg in 500 ml of saline or dextrose given I.V. infusion at the rate of 0.02 mg/ml.

ADR:

i. It splits to release cyanide. Larger doses may produce psychosis due to thiocyanate.
ii. Palpitation.
iii. Nervousness.
iv. Vomiting.
v. Perspiration.
vi. Pain abdomen.
vii. Weakness.
viii. Lactic acidosis (by released cyanide).

Available as 50 mg/5 ml.

TRADE NAME: SONIDE; PRUSIDE.

SODIUM STIBOGLUCONATE

Enlisted in Indian essential medicine list.

It is drug for kala-azar. It is pentavalent antimonial compound contains 1/3 of antimony by weight.

It is rapidly absorbed from I.M. injection site and excreted unchanged with urine. Repeat dose produces cumulation. Recently kala-razar of Bihar started showing resistance to it.

Dose: 20 mg/kg I.M. or I.V. × 20 to 30 days according to clinical response.

Available as 100 mg/ml in 30 ml vial.

ADR: Nausea, vomiting, metallic taste, cough, pain abdomen, pain at injected muscle, abscess, pancreatitis, liver and kidney damage, bone marrow depression, mental changes, shock and death.

SODIUM THIOSULFATE

Included both in WHO and Indian essential medicine list.

This is topically applied, weak fungistatic, particularly effective against *Malassezia furfur,* applied as 20% solution BD × 2-3 weeks for pityriasis versicolor.

Available as 20% solution.

TRADE NAME: KARPIN LOTION.

SODIUM VALPROATE

Enlisted in WHO and Indian essential medicine list.

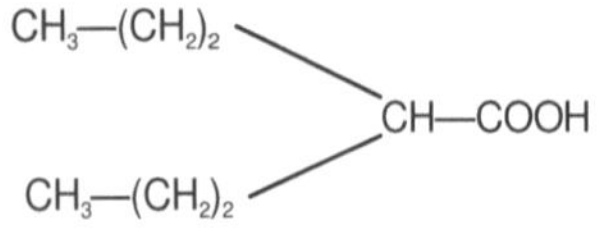

This is branched chain aliphatic carboxylic acid with broad spectrum anticonvulsant action acts by several mechanisms.

i. Prolonging frequency dependent Na channel inactivation.
ii. Weak attenuation of calcium mediated T current.
iii. Augments release of GABA and inhibitsdegradation of GABA.

It is orally absorbed, 90% protein bound, metabolized in liver (some are active) by oxidation and glucuronide conjugation and excreted with urine. Its anticonvulsant actions are long lasting.

ADR: Anorexia, vomiting, heart burn, drowsiness, ataxia, tremor, curling of hair, alopecia, rash, thrombocytopenia, rise in serum amino transaminase, fulminant hepatitis, spina bifida and other neural tube defects (if used during pregnancy).

Dose: 200 mg TDS upto 800 mg, 15-30 mg/kg/day.

Therapeutic Uses: Absence seizure, GTCS, SPS, CPS, mania and bipolar illness, prophylactic in migraine.

Drug Interactions: Increases plasma level of phenobarbitone, displaces phenytoin from plasma binding site and induces metabolism of carbamazepine. Use with clonazepam induces absence seizures.

Available as 200, 300, 500 mg tab; 200 mg/5 ml syr.

Co-ordination compound of valproic acid and sodium valproate is divalproex, marketed as diproex.

TRADE NAME: VALPARIN.

SPECTINOMYCIN

Included in WHO's essential medicine list.

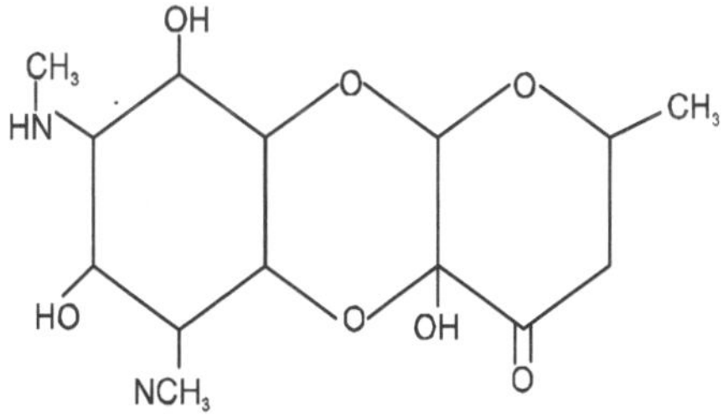

Spectinomycin is aminocyclitol antibiotic produced by *Streptomyces spectabilis*. It is therapeutically used for *N. gonococcal*urethritis, proctitis.

ADR: Pain at injection site, nausea, chills, fever, insomnia, urticaria, Hb % is decreased; raised serum alkaline phosphatase,

SGPT and BUN is increased. Safety of drugs in pregnancy and children is not established.

Dose: 2-4 g I.M. to be divided between two gluteal injection sites. Larger doses required for penicillin resistant cases.

Available as 2 and 4 g with 3.2 and 6.2 diluents.
TRADE NAME: TROBICIN.

SPIRONOLACTONE

WHO and Indian essential medicine enlisted drug.

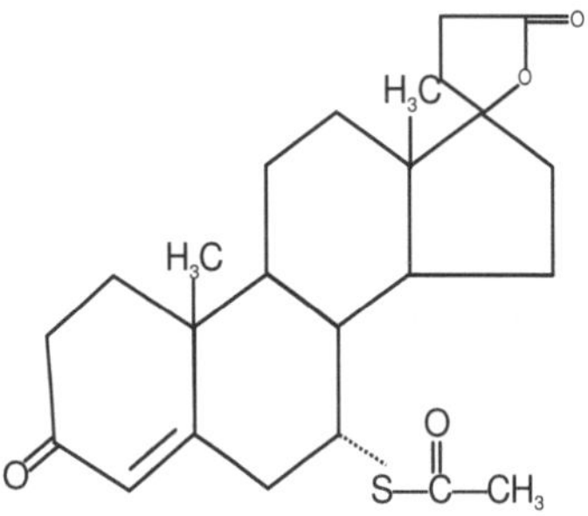

This is a potassium sparing diuretic, chemically a steroid related to mineralocorticoid aldosterone. It acts on distal tube and collecting duct by combining with intracellular mineralocorticoid receptors, which induces formation of aldosterone induced proteins to promote Na^+ resorption.

Orally absorbed (75%) plasma protein bound; metabolized in liver, some to cavrenone (active drug), undergoes enterohepatic circulation.

Dose: 25-50 mg BD to QD.

Therapeutic Uses: Edemas (Cirrhosis; Nephrotic syndrome) to counter the effect of thiazide's K^+ loss; hypertension; CCF.

ADR: Drowsiness, confusion, abdominal discomfort, hirsutism, gynaecomastia, impotence, menstrual irregularities, hyperkalemia, peptic ulcer.

Interaction: Aspirin blocks its action by inhibiting cavrenones, tubular secretion. It raises plasma digoxin level. Don't give K^+ simultaneously to avoid hyperkalemia.

Available as 25 and 100 mg tab.
TRADE NAME: ALDACTONE

STAVUDINE

Included both in WHO and Indian essential drug list.

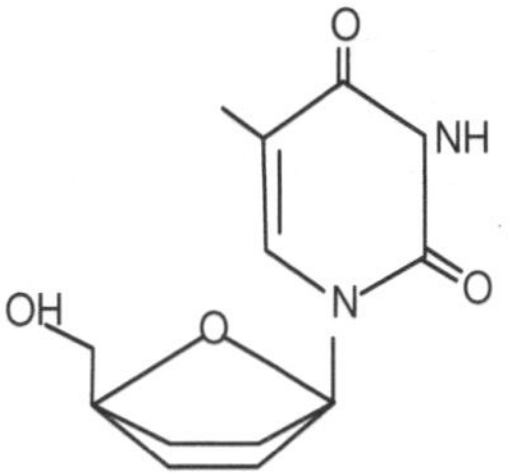

This nucleoside reverse transcriptase inhibitors, (NRTIs) is anti-HIV agent.

It is thymide analogue. Zudovudine antagonises, the effect of stavudine.

It is orally absorbed and rapidly metabolized.

ADR: Neuropathy, lipodystrophy, rarely pancreatitis.

Dose: 40 mg BD.

Available as 30 and 40 mg caps.

TRADE NAME: STAVIR; STAG.

STREPTOKINASE

Enlisted in WHO and Indian essential medicine list.

The source of streptokinase is *Beta Hemolytic streptococci group C. Per se* it is inactive, combines with circulating plasminogen to form activator complex which causes limited proteolysis of plasminogen to form plasmin. Antibodies present due to past infections inactivate considerable fractions of initial dose of streptokinase t/2 30-80 minutes.

It is antigenic and may cause hypersensitivity reactions and anaphylaxis if used for second time. Fever, hypotension, arrhythmia may accur. It is still used in India. Newer fibrinolytics are less likely to produce those effects.

Therapeutic Uses:

i. Myocardial infarction.
ii. Deep vein thrombosis.
iii. Pulmonary embolism.

Dose: For deep vein thrombosis and pulmonary embolism. 2.5 lac I.U., intravenous loading over ½ to 1 hour, followed by 1 lac I.U./ hour in 24 hours.

For myocardial infarction 7.5-15 lac I.U. unit I.V. over 1 hour.

Available as 2.5 lac, 7.5 lac and 15 lac I.U./vial.

TRADE NAME: STREPTASE; ESKINASE.

STREPTOMYCIN

Included both in WHO and Indian essential medicine list.

Streptomycin in the first drug effective against tuberculosis. It is obtained from *Streptomyces griseus.* Its spectrum includes H. ducreyi; *Brucella Y. pestis, F. tulareusis, Nocardia; C. granulomatis; M. tuberculosis.*

It binds 30 ribosomal subfraction and freeze initiation of proteins synthesis of bacteria.

It is highly ionized so not absorbed from G.I.T. excreted with urine without metabolism.

ADR: Vestibular toxicity, nephrotoxicity, hypersensitivity, rash, fever, exfoliative dermatitis, pain at injection site, paraesthesia.

Available as 0.75 gm and 1G power/vial. To be reconstituted before injection.

Dose: 0.75-1g O.D. I.M. for 7-10 days for acute infectious and for tuberculosis patient same dose up to 30-60 days.

TRADE NAME: AMBISTRYN.

SUCCINYL CHOLINE

Enlisted both in Indian and WHO's essential medicine list.

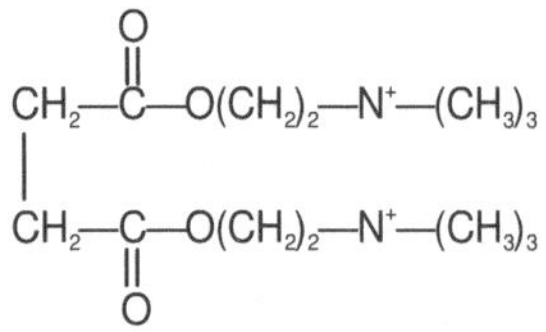

It is commonly used skeletal muscle relaxants for passing tracheal tube. It is brief acting because of rapid hydrolysis by cholinesterase. Used for intubation, laryngospasm, endoscopy, orthopaedic manipulation, electroconvulsive therapy.

ADR: Post operative apnea, fasciculation, change in BP, HR and arrhythmia, histamine release, hyperkalaemia due to K^+efflux, risk of regurgitation of gastric contents especially in obese and GERD patient.

Available as 50 mg/ml inj in 2 ml ampoule.

TRADE NAME: MIDARINE; SCOLINE.

SULFACETAMIDE

Included in Indian essential medicine list.

This sulfonamide derivative is available only for topical ophthalmic use. It is highly soluble compound yielding neutral solution and only mildly irritating to eye in concentration up to 30%.

It is used topically for conjunctivitis due to *Staph. aureus, D. pneumoniae; H. aegyptim; H. influenzae; N. catarrhalis, Cl. oculogenitalis.*

Available as 10, 20, 30% eye drop and 6% eye ointment.
TRADE NAME: LOCULA; ALBUCID.

SULFADIAZINE

Enlisted both in WHO and Indian essential medicine list.

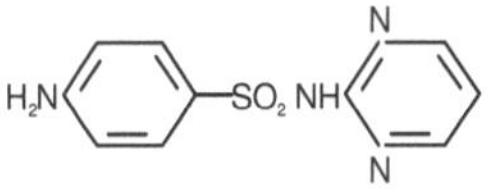

This sulfonamide derivative is used for U.T.I., prophylactically for recurrence of rheumatic fever and instilled topically on eye. It is no longer used because of large dose and alkalization of urine is required.

Dose: 2-4 g daily then 1 gm 6 hourly. For children 75 mg/kg body weight then 150 mg/kg daily in 4-6 divided doses. Topical 5% ointment.

For prophylactic to rheumatic fever 500 mg/day in weight below 30 kg and above that 1gm/day.

For trachoma adult 3 gm daily in divided dose or 100 mg/kg × 1 week then 60 mg/kg in four divided doses for 2 weeks.

ADR: Nausea, vomiting, epigastric pain, crystalluria rash, urticaria, photosensitization, kernicterus, hepatitis cool.

Available as 0.5 g tab; 0.5% oint.
TRADE NAME: SULFADIAZINE.

SULFADOXINE

Enlisted in WHO's essential medicine list.

It is ultra long sulfonamide because of high protein binding and slow renal excretion, so not suitable for acute pyogenic infection. Used for pneumocystis jiroveci pneumonia of AIDS; Toxoplasmosis and in combination with pyrimethamine in malaria.

SULFAMETHOXAZOLE

WHO enlisted essential medicine.

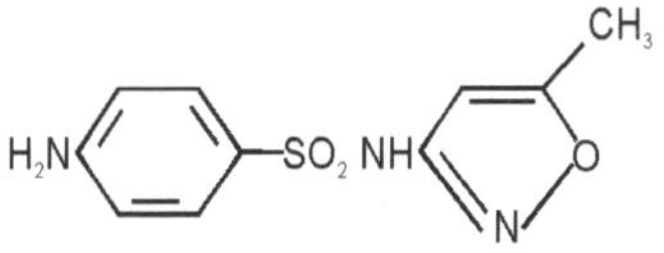

It is intermediate acting sulfonamide used for treating lower urinary tract infections by susceptible organism and for treating systemic infection by susceptible organism. It is combined with trimethoprim for the same purposes.

Its absorption and excretion of the unconjugated drug is slower therefore its blood level is excessive and it has greater tendency to produce crystalluria. Alkalization is unnecessary but adequate urinary output 1500 ml daily should be maintained.

Dose: 2 gm initially then 1 gm 2-3 times daily. Children over 2 months 60 mg/kg then half of this amount every twelve hourly.

Available as 500 mg/5 ml susp and 500 mg tab.

SULFASALAZINE

WHO and Indian essential medicine enlisted drug.

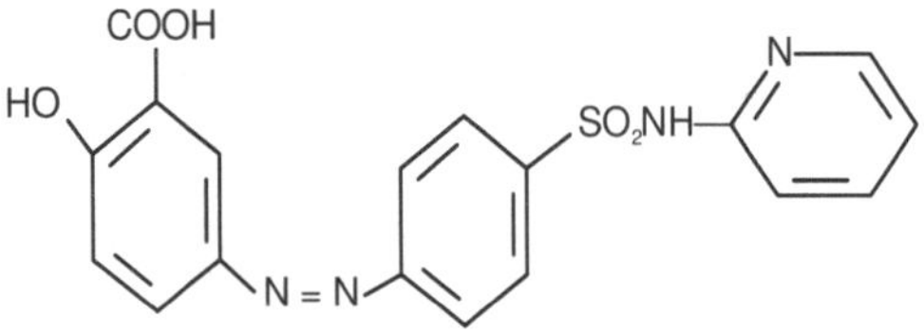

This sulfonamide derivative is a compound of sulfasalazine and 5 amino salicylic acid. It is used for:

i. Ulcerative colitis, Crohn's disease, diverticulitis.
ii. Rheumatoid arthritis.

It is poorly absorbed from ileum due to poor solubility. Its azo bonds split by colonic bacteria to release 5 amino salicylic acid, which exerts anti-inflammatory effects by inhibiting PG and LT production, cytokines, PAF, TNF α and NFKB.

Dose: For ulcerative colitis: 3-4 g/day for remission and 1.5-2 gm for maintenance.

Dose for rheumatoid arthritis 1-3 g/day in 2-3 divided doses.

Available as 0.5 g tab.

ADR: Headache, nausea, vomiting, fever, rash agranulocytosis. TRADE NAME: SAZO-EN.

SURAMIN

Included in WHO's essential medicine list.

This is a complexed derivative of urea used in the treatment and prophylaxis of trypanosomiasis and also used for onchocerciasis.

It is administered I.V. as it is not absorbed from G.I.T. and I.M. administration is painful. It is highly protein bound and may persist in plasma as long as 3 months. It does not cross BBB, so not effective in the encephalitis stages of these diseases.

ADR: Nausea, vomiting, colic, urticaria, shock, syncope, acute circulatory failure, allergy due to protein released by microfilariae (pruritis, rash), fever, oedema, burning and hyperesthesia of sole and feet, photophobia, iritis, lacrymation.

It is white powder soluble in water.

Dose: 10% solution in water for injection is used for onchocerciasis. Adults: 200-500 mg initially test the tolerance and then 1 gm weekly for 5 weeks. In children: 100 mg to test the tolerance and then 10-15 mg/kg body weight for 5 weeks.

In USA it is distributed from parasitic disease drug service.

TAMOXIFEN

It is enlisted both in WHO and Indian essential medicine lists.

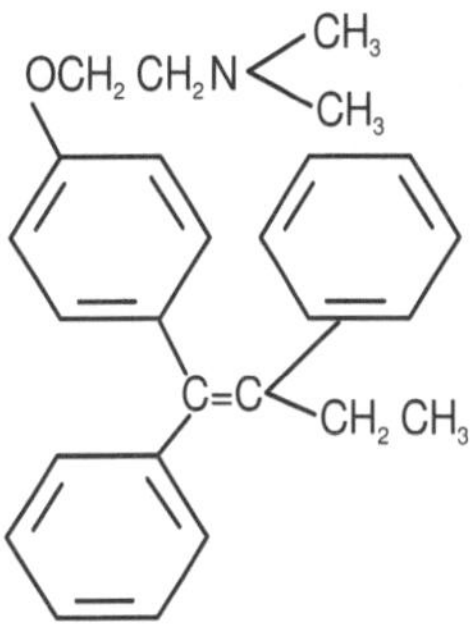

It is selective estrogen receptor modulator (SERM), competitive partial agonist inhibitor estradiol at the estrogen receptor. This is non steroidal in structure given orally. It is used in breast cancer patient in post menopausal women and for chemo-prevention in high risk women.

Hot flushes and inhibition of breast cancer reflects antioestrogenic action, since it is weak estrogenic to which manifest as endometrial proliferation, lowers Gn and prolactin level and improves bone density. It decreases LDL and cholesterol which adds to its benefits.

It is orally effective with biphasic plasma t/2 of 10 hours and 7 days which makes it long acting. It is excreted with bile.

Therapeutic Uses: ER +ve breast cancer of female, male breast cancer, male infertility as alternatine to clomiphene.

ADR: Vomiting, vaginal bleeding, hot flushes, thromboembolism, dermatitis, anorexia, depression, ocular changes, leukopenia.

Dose: 10-20 mg BD.

Available as 10 and 20 mg tabs.

TRADE NAME: MAMOFEN; TAMOXIFEN.

TENOFOVIR DISOPROXIL FUMARATE

Included in WHO essential medicine list.

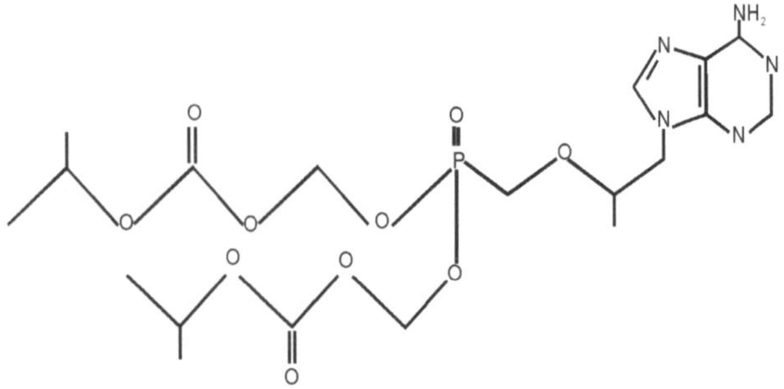

This NRT-I is acyclic nucleoside phosphate an analogs of adenosine, competitively inhibits HIV reverse transcriptase to produce chain termination after being incorporated into DNA.

It is orally absorbed which increases after fatty meal. Eliminated by glomerular filtration and secretion, so dose adjustment should be done in renal impaired patient.

Dose: 300 mg QDS.

ADR: Headache, asthenia, nausea, vomiting, diarrhea, flatulence, renal insufficiency.

Available as 300 mg tab.

TRADE NAME: VIREAD.

TERAZOSIN

It is enlisted in Indian essential medicine list.

It is reversible α_1 selective antagonist. It has high biological availability and longer t/2 of 12 hours or more. Chemically it is quinazoline derivative.

Uses: (i) Benign hyperplasia of prostrate, probably it has got an apoptosis promoting effect on prostrate too. (ii) Hypertension.

Dose: 2-10 mg OD.

Available as 1, 2, 5 mg tabs.

TRADE NAME: HYTRIN.

TERBUTALINE

Included in Indian essential medicine list.

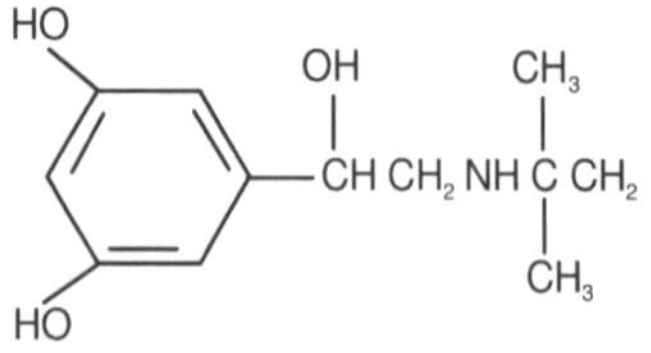

This β_2 agonist may be administered S/C or orally by inhalation. Inhaled terbutaline is popular as antiasthmatic.

ADR: Tremor, dizziness, nervousness, fatigue, tinnitus, palpitation. Arrhythmic, regular users should use inhaled steroids because it down regulates B receptor.

Therapeutic Uses:

i. Bronchial asthma, may be used as tocolytics.
ii. Hyperkalemic periodic paralysis because β agonist enhances K^+ uptake by muscle.

Dose: 5 mg oral, 0.25 S/C, 250 microgram by inhalation.

Available as 2.5, 5 mg tab, 3 mg/5 ml syr, 0.5 ml/ml inj: 250 µg/ metered dose.

TRADE NAME: BRICAREX; MISTHALER for inhalation.

TESTOSTERONE PROPIONATE

Enlisted in Indian essential medicine list.

It is used to develop or maintain secondary sexual character in male in androgen deficient patient. It is used perenterally for steady response but suitable for long term therapy. In older patient prostrate may enlarge to produce bladder neck obstruction. It is also used for palliative treatment of breast cancer in female. It may also be used perenterally for anabolic steroid.

Dose: I.M.10 to 25 mg biweekly for androgen deficiency; 50 to 100 mg bi to tri weekly for metastatic breast cancer in female. For anabolic effect 10-25 mg daily.

Buccal: Androgen deficient patient 5-20 mg daily in divided doses, post pubertal cryptorchism and hypogonadism. 15 mg daily in women to prevent post partum breast engorgement. 200 mg per day for androgen sensitive inoperable breast cancer.

Available as 25, 50 mg/ml injection. Buccal tablet 10 mg.

TRADE NAME: TESTOVIRAN ORETON.

TENTANUS TOXOID

Included in WHO and Indian essential medicine list.

Toxoids are prepared by modifying the bacterial exotoxins in such a way that their toxicity is lost but antigenicity is retained.

Tetanus toxoids are formalin treated exotoxins of tetanus bacilli. It may be fluid or adsorbed. The adsorbed toxoids provide better antibodies and it provides long acting immunity.

Dose: 0.5 ml I.M. or S/C.

For primary immunization 2 doses at 4-6 weeks gaps are given and booster after year and then every 10 years. The persons who are not immunized, it should be taken after any injury likely to introduce tetanus. Simultaneous administration of chloramphenicol interferes with antibody response.

Available as 0.5 ml amp or 10 ml vial.

ADR: Local erythema, pain, induration, fever, chill, malaise, paresis and other neurological complications are rare.

TETRACAINE

Included in WHO and Indian essential medicine lists.

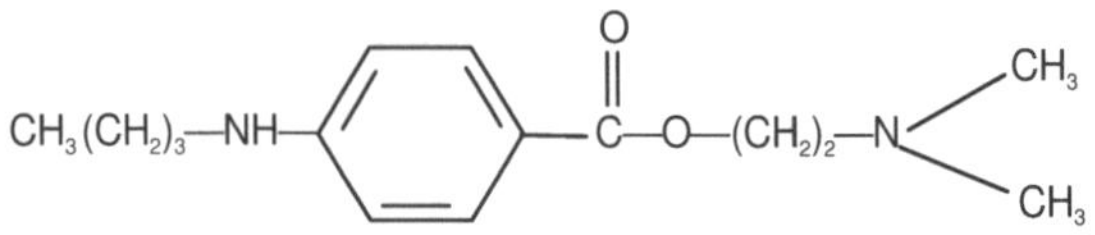

Tetracaine is a derivative of aminobenzoic acid (PABAester) used for surface, nerve block, infiltration, caudal and spinal anesthesia. It is approximately 10 times more potent and toxic to procaine and five to eight times more potent than cocaine when applied topically because of slow hydrolysis by pseudo-cholinesterase. Its use is generally restricted to eye, nose, throat, tracheobronchial tree and rarely for spinal or caudal anesthesia.

Dose: Maximum single dose 50 mg topically and 100 mg with adrenaline 1: 200000 by injection. Topical 0.5% as ointment or 1% as cream. Not more than 1 ounce for adults or ¼ ounce for children should be applied in 24 hours.

Nose and pharynx up to 4 ml of 1% solution. Don't use 20% solution.

Injection seldom used because of toxicity and slow onset of action if used 0.15% 0.25% with adrenaline 1:200000 (caudel 30 ml). Spinal 0.2 or 0.3% hyperbaric or 1% solution diluted with equal volume of 10% dextrose prepared for spinal anaesthesia. For saddle block (perineum 5 mg), for lower extremities and caesarean section 7-10 mg, for higher level and intra-abdominal surgery 12-15 mg.

Available as powder 20 mg; solution 0.2% with dextrose 6% in 2 ml container 0.3% with dextrose 6% 5 ml container (saddle block; perineal); 1% with NaCl 6.7mg and acetone sodium trisulfite 2 mg in 2 ml container.

Topical cream 1% in 1 ounce container; 0.5% ointment with menthol 5% white petroleum in one ounce container; 0.15% in 15 and 60 ml container; 2% in 30 and 120 ml container.
TRADE NAME: PONTOCAINE.

TETRACYCLINE

It is both in WHO and Indian essential medicine lists.

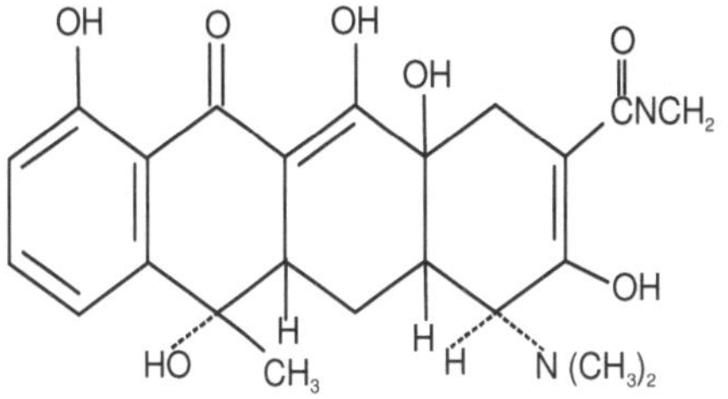

It was introduced in 1955. It is an antibiotic with four cyclic rings, all are obtained from soil actinomycetes. It is available as base HCL salt and PO_4 complex. It is bacteriostatic, binds to 305 ribosomes of susceptible organism to inhibit peptide chain. Resistance occurs slowly, cross resistance seen with different members of tetracycline except minocycline. Partial cross resistant seen with chloramphenicol.

Used for chlamydial, non specific urethritis, lymphogranuloma venereum, granuloma inguinale, atypical pneumonia, cholera, brucellosis, plague, relapsing fever by Borrelia recurrentis, Rickettsial infection (Typhus, Rocky mountain spotted fever, Q-fever.

It is second choice for listeria; Gonorrhoea (if resistant or allergic to penicillin); Chlamydia pneumoniae; Chancroid; Tularemia if resistant to first drug.

Other Uses: COPD, community acquired pneumonia, Amoebiasis, Acne vulgaris; UTI.

Precaution: It should not be used in pregnancy and lactation, with diuretics, in hepatic and renal insufficiency. Don't give after expiry date or intrathecally and in children below 12 years.

ADR: A. Nausea, vomiting, diarrhoea, epigastric pain, if given I.M. thrombophlebitis, pain.

B. Dose related: Liver damage, renal damage, phototoxicity, antianabolic effects, increased intracranial pressure, diabetes insipidus,vestibular toxicity.

C. Hypersensitivity.

D. Super infection.

Available as 250 mg, 500 mg cap, 3% skin ointment, 1% eye/ ear drop.

TRADE NAME: HOSTACYCLINE; RESTECLIN.

THEOPHYLLINE COMPOUNDS

Enlisted in Indian essential medicine list.

Preparations available and doses.

i. Theophylline anhydrous, poorly water soluble. Dose: 100-300 mg TDS; 15 mg/kg/day.

Theolong 100, 200 mg SR.

ii. Aminophylline discussed earlier.

iii. Hydroxyethyl theophylline (Etophylline 80% theophylline). It is water soluble can be given I.M. or I.V. not S/C; oral 250 mg, I.M. or I.V. Available as deriphylline 100 mg tab; 300 mg SR tab, 220 mg/2 ml inj.

iv. Choline theophyllinate 250-500 mg orally.
Available as choliphylline 125 mg cap, 125 mg/5 ml elixir.

v. Theophylline ethanolate of piperazine 250-500 mg oral or I.V.
Available as cardiphyllate 80 mg/5 ml. elixir; Etophylate 125 mg/5 ml syr.

vi. Doxyphylline is long acting methyl – xanthine.

Dose: 400 mg OD.

Available as Oxypur.

Use:

i. Bronchial asthma.
ii. COPD.
iii. Apnoea in premature infants.
iv. In myasthenia some improvement is found with theophylline compounds.

THIAMINE

Enlisted in WHO and Indian essential medicine lists.

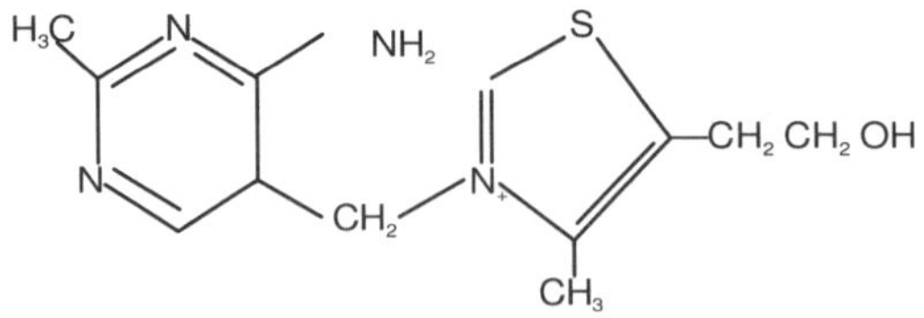

Vitamin B_1 or thiamine hydrochloride is widely distributed, is an essential co-enzyme for carbohydrate metabolism. It is colourless crystalline containing pyrimidine and thiazole ring. Present in outer layer of cereals, pulses, green vegetables, eggs, meats and nuts.

It is absorbed by active transport. It is converted in body as thiamine pyrophosphate and acts in decarboxylation of ketoacids, hexose monophosphate shunts.

Daily requirements 0.3 mg/1000 kcal. It is also involved in neuromuscular transmission. Tea contains thiamine antagonist. Pyrithiamine and oxythiamine are thiamine antagonist.

Thiamine deficiency occurs with alcoholism and malnutrition may produce:

i. Wernicke's encephalopathy (symptoms are: ophthalmoplegia, ataxia, polyneuropathy, mental disorientation).
ii. Korsakoff's syndrome (confabulatory psychosis).
iii. Dry beriberi (numbness, tingling, hyperesthesia, wrist drop,foot drop; loss of apetite, constipation).
iv. Wet beriberi: Palpitation, breathlessness, high output, cardiac failure, protein deficiency.

Therapeutic Uses:

i. Prophylactically (2-10 mg / day) as infants, chroni diarrhoea, perenteral nutrition.
ii. Beriberi (dry and wet).
iii. Alcohol intoxication.
iv. Hyperemesis gravidarum, anorexia, obstinate constipation.

Available as: Oral Thiamine HCl: 10, 25, 50, 100, 250 mg tabs; injection 100 mg/ml in 1, 10, 20 and 30 ml containers.

THIACETAZONE + ISONIAZID

Included in Indian essential medicine list.

It was discarded in the west because of hapatotoxicity but in India thiacitazone is used with INH for oral use as a substitute of PAS because of low toxicity. It is low efficacy tuberculostatic drug and delays development or resistance to isoniazid, streptomycin and ethambutol. Thiacetazone is excreted unchanged in urine.

ADR: Thiacetazone, Hepatitis, Stevens-Johnson syndrome, exfoliative dermatitis, bone marrow depression, anorexia, loose motion, abdominal discomfort. Thiacetazone produces serious toxicities to HIV patient.

Thiacetazone and INH tablet N.F. contains 50 mg of thiacetazone and 100 mg of INH.

Dose: 3 tab daily for adults.

THIOPENTAL SODIUM

Included in Indian essential medicine list.

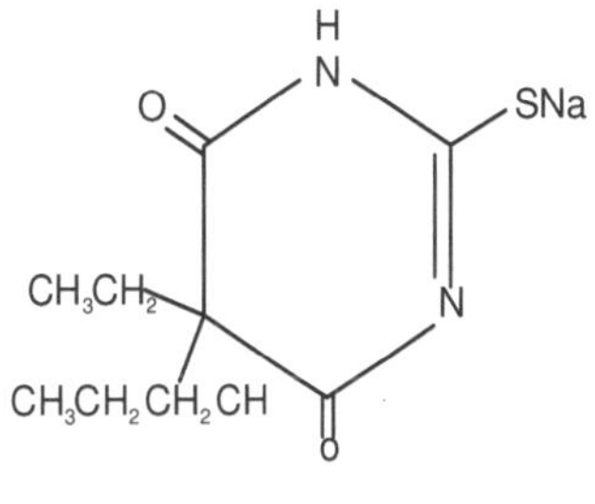

This rapid, potent hypnotic is useful for inducing general anesthesia. Its analgesic property is poor, so once the patient is unconscious anesthesia can be maintained by increasing or by dilute I.V. infusion or by supplementing nitrous oxide. It may be given rectally as basal anesthetic in children.

Dose: 3-5 mg/kg as 2.5% produces unconsciousness in 15-20 seconds. It is metabolized in liver. It has weak muscle relaxant, so addition of neuromuscular blocker and narcotic analgesics may require depending on the type of surgery.

It is rapidly taken up by fat cells from there it is gradually released.

ADR: Yawning, cough, laryngospasm, respiratory depression, BP may fall, extravasation may slough the skin, post anesthetic nausea, vomiting, CNS depression (patient should not be allowed to leave without an attendant), acute intermittent porphyria.

Available as 0.5, 1 gm powder. Use fresh.

Therapeutic Uses:

i. Intravenous anaesthesia.
ii. Rapid control of convulsion.
iii. Psychiatric patient.
iv. Narcoanalysis of criminals acts by knocking off the guarding.

TRADE NAME: PENTOTHAL; INTRAVAL SODIUM.

TIMOLOL

It is enlisted in WHO and Indian essential medicine lists.

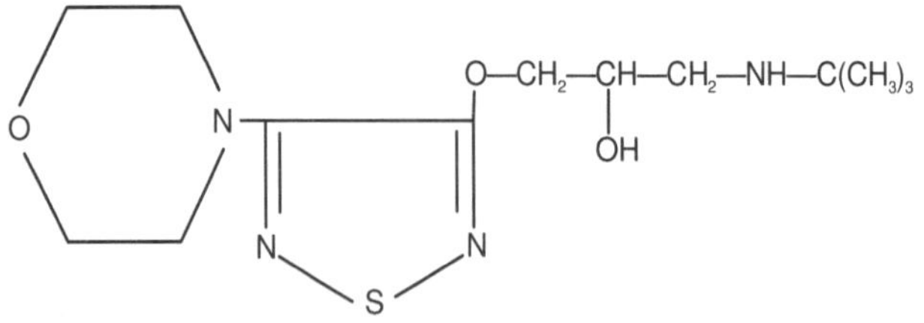

Timolol is nonselective β blocker (i.e. β_1 and β_2 blocker) used for decreasing intra ocular pressure of glaucoma and does not possess local anaesthetic or intrinsic sympathomimetic property. It decreases intra ocular tension smoothly and it is well sustained. 30% of open angle glaucoma needs additional medicine because timolol fails to achieve desired level of intra ocular tension.

Available as 0.25% and 0.5% drops. Dose is B.D.

It may precipitate bronchial asthma.

Therapeutic Uses:

i. Hypertension.
ii. CCF.
iii. Migraine prophylaxis.
iv. Open angle glaucoma and intra ocular hypertension.

TRADE NAME: GLUCOMOL; LOPRES.

TINIDAZOLE

Included in Indian essential medicine list.

This nitroimidazole derivative is efficacious congener of metronidazole. The major differences are: Metabolism is slower so long acting and ADR of nausea, vomiting and metallic taste are slower.

Therapeutic Uses:

i. Amoebiasis 2 g OD × 3 days (children 30-50 mg/day).
ii. Trichomoniasis 2 g single dose or 0.6 g × 7 days.
iii. Giardiasis: Dose is same as trichomoniasis.
iv. Anaerobic infection.
   a. Prophylactic: 2 gm single dose before infra umbilical or colorectal surgery.
   b. Therapeutic: 2 g followed by 0.5 g BD × 5 days.
v. H. pylori infection: 500 mg BD × 2 weeks with triple combination.

Available as: 300, 500, 1000 mg tab; 800 mg/400 ml I.V. infusion.

TRADE NAME: TINIBA; FASIGYN.

TRICLABENDAZOLE

Enlisted in WHO's essential medicine list.

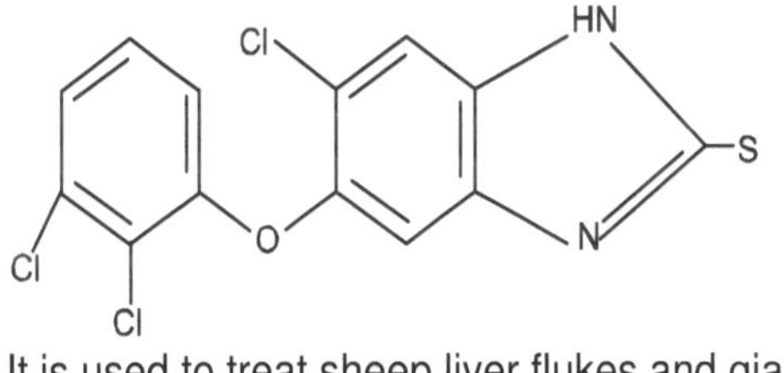

It is used to treat sheep liver flukes and giant liver flukes and other flatworm infection.

Available as 250 mg tab.

Dose: 10 mg/kg orally × 2 days.

It probably works by immobilizing the worm and it dies.

TRADE NAME: FASINEX.

TRIFLUPERAZINE

It is enlisted in Indian essential medicine list.

This antipsychotic drug is phenothiazine derivative with piperazine side chain.

It is orally absorbed.

Dose: 2-20 mg/day with antiemetic properties and severe extrapyramidal effects.

Available as 1-5 mg tabs.

It has minimal autonomic actions. Sedation, hypotension and seizure threshold is not significantly lowered. It is less likely to cause jaundice.

TRADE NAME: TRINICAM; NEOCALM.

TRIHEXYPHENIDYL

It is enlisted in Indian essential medicine list.

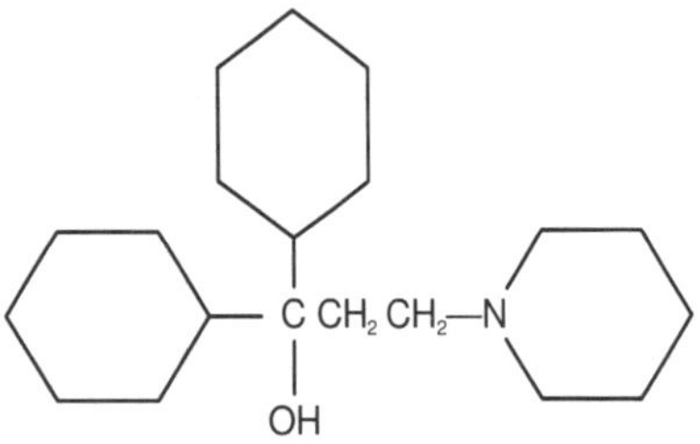

This durg is centrally acting anticholionergic used for parkinsonism idiopathic or post encephalopathic.

Dose start with 2 mg TDS and then increase gradually till therapeutic concentration is achieved. For durg induced parkinsonism dose is 1mg and if symptoms are not controlled with few hours, it is increased.

Available as 2 mg tab.

TRADE NAME: PACITANE; PARBENZ.

TRIMETHOPRIM

It is included in essential medicine list of both India and WHO.

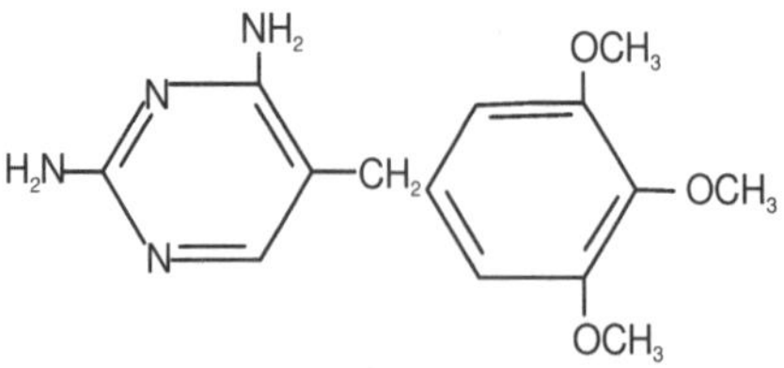

Dose: 100 mg - 200 mg BD; children, 6 mg/kg/day.

Therapeutic Uses: UTI, prostritis.

Other details of the drug is discussed with cotrimoxazole.

TROPICAMIDE

Enlisted both in WHO and Indian essential medicine lists.

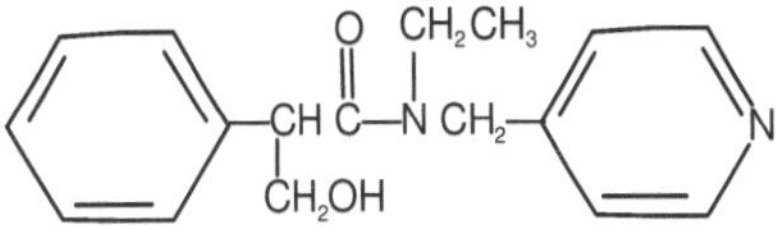

It is effective mydriatic and cycloplegic with rapid and short duration of action.

Therapeutic Uses:

Aid to refraction, ophthalmoscopy and retinal photography.

Dose: 1% solution are instilled in 5 minutes apart 2 drops produces maximal cycloplegia in 20-30 minutes, 0.5% solution produces pupillary dilatation in 20-50 minutes, the residual paralysis persists for seven hours. It rarely produces adverse reaction on topical application.

Available as 0.5 and 1% eye drops.

TRADE NAME: OPTIMIDE; TROMIDE.

TUBERCULIN PURIFIED PROTEIN DERIVATIVE

It is included in WHO and Indian essential medicine lists.

It is used for diagnosis of tuberculosis. It is slightly more refined tuberculin (which is prepared by autoclaving or boiling tubercle bacilli concentrated 10 fold by steam bath and filtering off that debris). PPD was first prepared by Seibert. Mol wt about 10000.

Solutions of PPD for Mantoux testing are available as dilution of 1:10000, 1:1000, 1:100 called 1,10,100 I.U. in the injected dose of 0.1 mg 1 ml. 1 ml. of PPD containing 5 I.U. in injected subcutaneously in volar aspect of skin of forearm in those suspected of tuberculosis. The site of inoculation is palpated after 72 hours. For firm induration 10 mm or more is said to be positive, 5-9 mm is doubtful. Accompanying erythema is ignored. If the test is negative, it may be repeated with 100 I.U.

TYPHOID VACCINE

It is enlisted in WHO's essential medicine list.

This is a sterile suspension of S.typhi and paratyphi bacillus. Each ml contains 1×10^9 S.typhi and 7.5×10^8 each of S. paratyphi A and B in 5 and 10 ml vial.

Dose: 0.5 ml S/C 2 to 3 injections in every 2-4 weeks and booster every 2-3 years.

Local tenderness, fever, malaise may occur. The paratyphoid added to typhoid vaccine seems to be ineffective and gives rise to adverse reactions more. It is 70% effective in preventing enteric fever for one year.

UREA

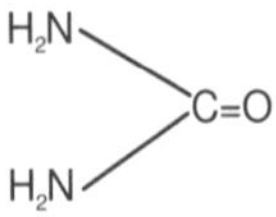

Urea when applied in the concentration 5-20% as cream/ointment acts as humectant because of its hygroscopic and water retaining properties. It softens and solubilizes keratin to remove hyperkeratinized skin lesions (viz. Icthyosis, lichen planus).

30% urea acts as diuretic, given I.V. acts as diuretic but not used because of its disadvantages.

UROKINASE

Urokinase is fibrinolytics or thrombolytics used to lyse thrombi or clots to recanalize the occluded vessels. This enzyme was isolated from human urine, now prepared from cultured human kidney cells. It activates plasminogen. it is non antigenic. Its t/2 10-15 minutes.

Available as 2.5, 5 and 10 lac I.U. per vial.

Dose for myocardial infection: 2.5 lac I.U. over 10 minutes followed by 5 lac I.U. over next one hour or 6000 I.U./min upto 2 hours. If recanalization has occurred. It is generally used who is exposed to streptokinase earlier.

For venous thrombosis and pulmonary embolism: 4400 I.U.over 10 minutes then 4400 I.U. per hour for 12 hours.

Fever, hypotension and allergic reactions are rare.

VANCOMYCIN

Obtained from *Streptomyces orientalis*. It is glycopeptides with mol. wt of 1500. Effective against gram positive bacteria particularly MRSA, *Strep viridans, Enterococcus, Cl. difficile*. It acts by inhibiting bacterial cell wall synthesis.

Its absorption from G.I.T. is poor, only used orally for treatment of enterocolitis due to *Cl. difficile* otherwise given I.V. It is widely distributed in body, mostly excreted by glomerular filtration. It cannot be excreted by haemodialysis.

Therapeutic Uses: Sepsis, endocarditis caused by MRSA, Pseudomembranous enterocolitis.

ADR: Chills, fever, phlebitis, red man or red neck syndrome due to release of histamine, which can be prevented by prolonging infusion time or infusion interval.

Available as 150 mg tab or 500 mg/vial.

Dose for enterocolitis: 0.125 - 0.250 mg 6 hourly orally. For other infections 30 mg/kg/day in two or three divided doses.

VARICELLA VACCINE

Varicella vaccine is lyophilized live attenuated OKa strain of varicella zoster virus. It is grown in human diploid culture. A single dose gives protection for 10 years.

Dose: 0.5 ml S/C single dose for children below 12 years. Children above 12 years requires 2 doses in 6-12 weeks apart.

Contraindicated in pregnancy, lymphocytopenia within one month of measles vaccination. Local maculopapular rash, fever may occur as ADR.

VECURONIUM

This skeletal muscle relaxant is included in essential medicine list of WHO.

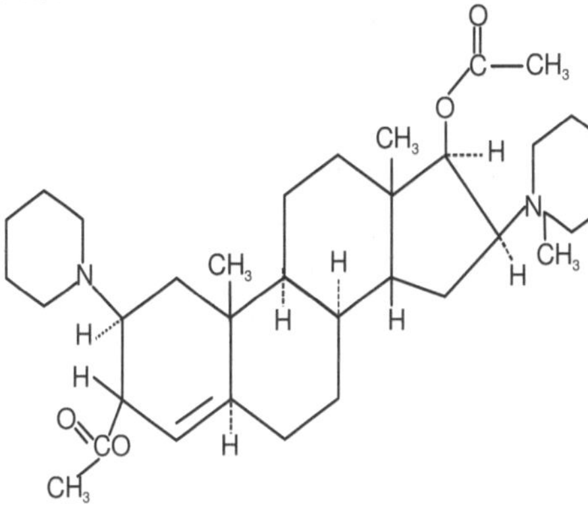

It is short acting because of rapid distribution and metabolism comparative to pancuronium. It is non-depolarising competitive neuromuscular blocking agent. Its recovery is generally spontaneous.

C.V.S. stability is better. It does not release histamine or block autonomic ganglia.

Available as 4 mg amp with 1 ml solvents. It is mostly eliminated by liver (70-90%) and kidney. It is commonly used skeletal muscle relaxant.

VERAPAMIL

It is included in WHO and Indian essential medicine lists.

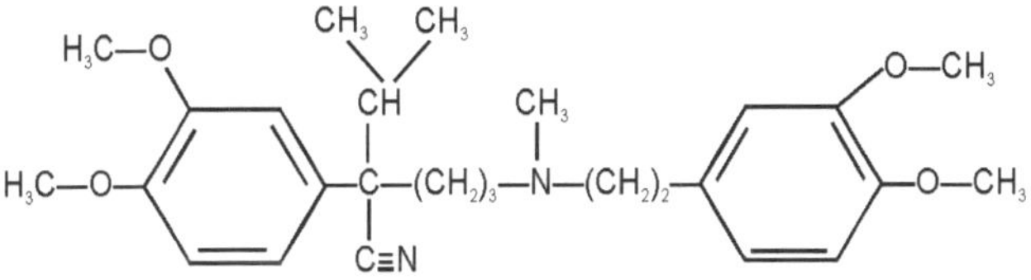

It is a calcium channel blocker (blocks L type ca channel). It also dilates arterioles and has some alpha adrenergic blocking action.

Therapeutic Uses:

i. Paroxysmal supraventricular tachycardia.
ii. To control ventricular rate in AF.
iii. Antianginal.

Available as 40 and 80 mg tab, 5 mg/2 ml injection.

Dose: 40-160 mg TDS oral or slow I.V. 5 mg.

ADR: Nausea, constipation, bradycardia, occasionally hypotension, contraindicated to heart block 2nd and 3rd degree.

Interaction: Do not give with β blocker, quinidine or disopyramide. It increases plasma digoxin level by decreasing its excretion.

VINBLASTINE

It is included in WHO and Indian essential medicine lists.

This plant alkaloid is obtained from periwinkle plant *Vinca rosea.*

It inhibits tubulin polymerization and disruption of assembly of microtubules and arrest of cell division in M phase of cell cycle.

Nausea, vomiting, bone marrow suppression, alopecia, vesication may occur.

Uses: Hodgkin and non-Hodgkin's lymphoma, breast cancer, germ cell cancer.

Dose: 0.1 -0.2 mg/kg I.V. weekly.

Available as 10 mg/vial injection.

VINCRISTINE

Included in WHO and Indian essential medicine lists.

It is a plant alkaloid obtained from *Vinca rosea.* It is also mitotic spindle poison acts on cell cycles M phase.

It is used with prednisolone for remission and induction of ALL. Also used for Hodgkin and non-Hodgkin's lymphoma, multiple myeloma, rhabdomyosarcoma, neuroblastoma, Ewing sarcoma, Wilm's tumour.

ADR: Neuropathy, orthostatic hypotension, sphincter problem, cranial nerve palsy, paralytic ileus, SIADH, myelosuppression, alopecia.

Available as 1 mg/vial.

Dose: 1.5 mg/sq meter.

VITAMIN B_{12} (CYANOCOBALAMINE)

Vitamin B_{12} are complex cobalt containing compounds of diet. Its daily requirement is 1-3 μgm in pregnancy and lactation it is 3-5 μgm. It is available in liver, kidney, egg yolk, meat, cheese. Commercially it is obtained from *Streptomyces griseus* by product of streptomycin. Its metabolic functions are as following:

a. Conversion of homocysteine to methionine.
b. Purine and pyrimidine synthesis.
c. Malonic acid is converted to succinic acid in its presence.
d. Methionine is converted to S-adenosyl methionine.
e. Essential for cell multiplication and growth.

Its deficiency occurs in pernicious anemia due to intrinsic factor deficiency, gastrectomy, malabsorption, blind loop syndrome, nutritional deficiency, pregnancy and lactation due to increased demand.

Deficiency manifest as:

i. Megaloblastic anaemia, glossitis, epethelial damage.
ii. Subacute combined degeneration of spinal cord.

Therapeutic Uses:

i. In deficiency states.
ii. Tobacco amblyopia.

ADR: Anaphylactoid reaction may occur if given I.V. otherwise safe.

Available as:

a. Cyanocobalabmine 35 μg/5 ml injection.
b. Hydroxycobalamine 500-1000 μg/ml injection.
c. Methylcobalamine 0.5 mg tab.

VITAMIN D_3 (ERGOCALCIFEROL)

It is included in WHO and Indian essential medicine lists.

It increases calcium absorption from intestine. It enhances tubular reabsorption of calcium in the kidney.

Its deficiency manifest as ricket in children and osteomalacia in adults where organic matrix osteoid formation is normal.

Hypervitaminosis of vitamin D may occur due to chronic ingestion which manifest as hypercalcaemia, polyuria, fatigue, albuminuria, ectopic calcium deposition, renal stone, hypertension. It is treated with withholding Vit D, low calcium diet, plenty of fluids and corticosteroids.

It is compared to hormone. In circulation it binds to α globulin and stored in body in adipose tissue, hydroxylated in liver to become active and inactive. Metabolites are excreted in bile mainly.

Preparations:

i. Calciferol (Gelatin capsules 25000-50000 IU/cap).
ii. Cholecalciferol as granules or oily solution for injection.
iii. Calcitriol 0.25-1 μg orally daily or on alternate day.

WARFARIN SODIUM

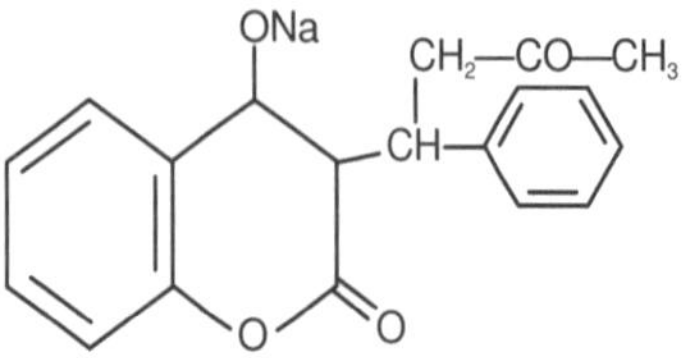

- Wisconsin
- Alumni
- Foundation
- With "arin" from coumarin.

Mechanism of Action: It blocks the gamma carboxylation of glutamate residues of prothrombin and factors VII, IX and X, i.e., Vitamin K dependent factors. It acts on vivo. Racemic warfarin is most popular anticoagulants. R form is less potent.

Available as 1, 2, 5 mg tab.

Its t/2 is 36-48 hours. Loading dose 10-15 mg. Maintenance dose is 2-10 mg. Its therapeutic effect starts when clotting factors synthesis are reduced to 40-50%. Alopecia, dermatitis, diarrhea may occur as ADR. Prothombin time should be assessed to adjust dose.

Treatment of Warfarin Bleeding:

i. Withhold warfarin.
ii. Fresh blood or fresh frozen plasma to supply clotting factors immediately.
iii. Vitamin as specific antidote.

Indications:

i. Prophylaxis and treatment of deep vein thrombosis, pulmonary embolism, TIA, HIP surgery.
ii. Prosthetic heart valves to prevent recurrent thromboembolism.

Drug Interactions:

i. Newer cephalosporins cause hypoprothrombinaemia and have additive effect with warfarin.
ii. Aspirin: Additive effects due to aspirin's antiplatelet effects and hypoprothrombinemic effects.
iii. Protein bound drugs (long acting sulfonamide probenecid etc) displaces it from protein binding so dose adjustment is required.
iv. Phenytoin and tolbutamide, erythromycin, cimetidine inhibit warfarin's metabolism.

XYLOMETAZOLINE

It is included in national list of essential medicines of India (2003).

It is α (alpha agonist), used as topical application 0.05 to 0.1% diluted applied on nose. After congestion is claimed to be less.

Prolong use impairs mucosal ciliary function. Atropic rhinitis, anosmia etc may occur due to prolong vasoconstriction. It may be absorbed from nasal mucosa to produce rise in BP, CNS depression. Should not be used with patient receiving MAO inhibitors and in hypertensives.

Ideal Nasal Decongestants

i. It should produce prompt, prolong and reliable action.
ii. Should not produce tachyphylaxis, local irritation, after congestion and should not damage the nasal cilia.

ZIDOVUDINE (AZT)

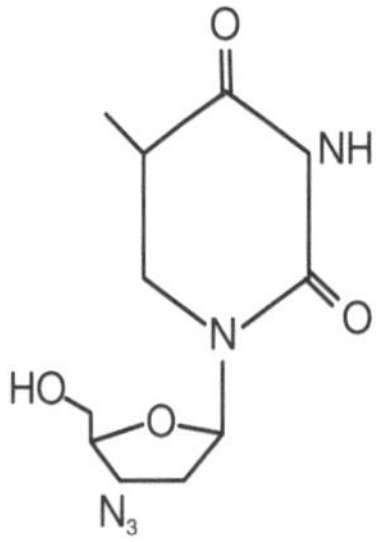

It belongs to nucleoside and nucleotide reverse transcriptase inhibitor, effective against anti retroviral agents. Chemically azidothymidine (AZT) a deoxythmidine analogue.

Dose: 200 mg TID or 300 mg BID. Adjust in renal insufficiency.

It is orally absorbed, distributed in most tissues including CSF. Excreted with urine after glucuronidation.

Efficacy proved in HIV associated dementia, thrombocytopenia. It may be given to pregnant lady with HIV infection.

Dose: 100 mg 5 times a day or during labor 1 mg/kg/hour by I.V. infusion. Resistance may occur.

ADR: Myelosuppression, neutropenia, macrocytic anaemia, G.I. intolerance, headache, insomnia hypopigmentation of nails, myopathy, vaginal neoplasm.

Drug Interactions

i. Probenecid, phenytoin, fluconazole, atovaquone, valproic acid increase its level.
ii. Zidovudine may decrease phenytoin level.

iii. Myelosuppressive drugs increases hematological toxicity on co-administration.

ZIDOVUDINE + LAMIVUDINE + NEVIRAPINE

This fixed drug combinations have been approved by WHO for HIV infection. Lamivudine is NRTI.

Dose: 150 mg BID.

Nevirapine is non-nucleoside reverse transcriptase inhibitor NNRTI. Dose 1250 mg BID.

ZINC-OXIDE

Enlisted in Indian essential medicine list.

Zinc oxide is a component of calamine lotion. It acts as a mild astringent. Calamine is zinc oxide with small amount of ferric oxide. It is insoluble in water. It when applied over skin acts as an antiseptic, dermal protective, adsorbent.

ZINC-SULFATE

Included in WHO and Indian essential medicine lists.

It is water soluble. 0.1-1% are used as eye wash, ear drops (zinc and boric acid drops). It decreases perspiration if applied on skin. Zinc sulfate with sulfurated potash is used for acne and impetigo.